Showdown
with Diabetes

Showdown with Diabetes

DEB BUTTERFIELD

Foreword by David E. R. Sutherland, M.D., Ph.D.

W. W. Norton & Company

New York London

Copyright © 1999 by Insulin-Free World Foundation

For information about permission to reproduce selections from this book,
write to Permissions, W. W. Norton & Company, Inc., 500 Fifth Avenue,
New York, NY 10110

The text and display of this book is composed in Simoncini Garamond
Desktop composition by Gina Webster
Manufacturing by the Quebecor Companies, Inc.
Book design by Chris Welch

Library of Congress Cataloging-in-Publication Data
Butterfield, Deb.
Showdown with diabetes / Deb Butterfield ; foreword by David E. R. Sutherland.
p.   cm.
ISBN 0-393-04753-9
1. Butterfield, Deb—Health. 2. Diabetes—Patients—United States—Biography.
3. Pancreas—Transplantation—Patients—United States—Biography.
4. Kidneys—Transplantation—Patients—United States—Biography.
5. Diabetes—Treatment. I. Title.
RC660.B83   1999
362.1'96462'0092—dc21
[b]   99–19651
CIP

W. W. Norton & Company, Inc., 500 Fifth Avenue, New York, N.Y. 10110
www.wwnorton.com

W. W. Norton & Company Ltd., 10 Coptic Street, London WC1A 1PU

1 2 3 4 5 6 7 8 9 0

To my donor, Ann, who in her passing gave me health

Contents

Foreword

by David E. R. Sutherland, M.D., Ph.D.

Showdown with Diabetes relates two odysseys. The first is the personal odyssey of Deb Butterfield as she traverses a road with diabetes from a condition to a disease, degenerating into disability, and finally a successful uphill battle to insulin independence with a pancreas transplant. The second, a story within a compelling story, is the epochal one of advances in the understanding and treatment of diabetes in this century, the misconceptions of how diabetes affects individuals, and the limitations of our current therapeutic options.

I met Deb for the first time at the University of Minnesota Hospital pretransplant clinic in 1993, where she came as a candidate for a pancreas-kidney transplant to treat insulin-dependent diabetes mellitus. In spite of her advanced diabetic complications, she sat with a big optimistic smile as we discussed the mechanics of a double organ retransplant. Deb is typical and atypical of the diabetic patients I have treated with pancreas transplants over the years. She is typical in that, like most people who ultimately succeed in achieving their objective of insulin independence, she fought through layers of naysayers. Yet Deb is atypical in her extraordinary ability to express her feelings, to strip away the myths surrounding diabetes, transplants, and related matters, and to rally others to action to improve the lot of diabetics, both *today* and tomorrow.

I have been involved with transplants for people with diabetes for more than twenty years. A small cadre of transplant surgeons took on the challenge in the 1970s, and now, in the 1990s, approximately eleven thousand pancreas transplants have been done worldwide. It is the only treatment that consistently—in nearly 90 percent of the cases—induces continuously normal blood-sugar levels without the need for insulin, meal planning, or blood-glucose monitoring.

Only one percent of the cells in the pancreas, the islet cells, are involved with insulin production. Thus, even as pancreas transplantation was evolving into a highly successful treatment of diabetes, an army of investigators has been researching how to achieve insulin independence with a technology requiring only a simple, lasting injection of islets. This, too, can work, but currently only 10 percent of islet recipients have become insulin independent. Both pancreas and islet transplants require the use of drugs to prevent them from being rejected by the immune system. Much of today's research to cure diabetes is directed at the longer-term prospect of eliminating the need for these drugs. *Show-down with Diabetes* addresses today's treatment choices and sheds light on the decisions that diabetic people must make as to whether to forego actual advances in treatment while waiting for the promise of others that may be "just around the corner."

Through her personal story and her analysis of the benefits and shortcomings of insulin in Part 2 of her book, Deb provides insights into the paradox of how advances in technology to manage diabetes have shifted the responsibility for the disease from the ailment to the person who has it. Of course, tight control may delay or decrease the probability of developing secondary complications of diabetes. However, to attempt this level of control, the diabetic individual must rigidly adhere to a schedule of medical management that is incompatible with the roller coaster we call life. I agree with Deb: The burden of living with diabetes is often grossly underestimated by even the doctors and nurses directly involved. It is more than finger pricks, injections, and meal planning. It is living in the shadow of the debilitating, long-term complications of the disease—and of knowing that even one's best efforts may be insufficient to prevent them.

The objectives of modern research should be to free diabetic people from this burden. Prevention of diabetes in the first place is the ideal. Failing that, transplantation of insulin-producing cells, either within an intact pancreas or as an injection of cells, must do. Better yet would be to circumvent the need for ongoing drug therapies by regenerating the ability of a person's native islets to produce insulin. But, as *Show-*

down with Diabetes explains, right now only pancreas trans-plants are a reality, and although they cannot cure diabetes, they are a better treatment for many diabetics than intensive insulin management. Pancreas transplantation is wholly underutilized. It works. And until something better comes along, labile diabetics and those prone to complications—if not any diabetic patient—certainly should consider it. Deb's experience of living with diabetes and of achieving insulin independence with a pancreas transplant highlights the crux of today's treatment choices—do the side effects of immuno-suppression exceed the problems of diabetes? It sheds light on the judgments, probabilities, and informed consent inher-ent in these choices.

Deb's mission is not simply to tell her story; it is to create awareness of what diabetes really means to the individuals afflicted and what solutions are available now, and to indicate where research is leading us. From *Showdown with Diabetes* to her work as the executive director of the Insulin-Free World Foundation, the nonprofit organization she founded, Deb wants what we all want—an insulin-free world. She wants the portions of her story that are common anecdotes—the uncertainties, complications, and restrictions of dia-betes—to be uncommon anecdotes. She wants those elements of her story that are uncommon—achieving insulin independence—to be common.

Preface

Chronic illness is at the same time a personal misfortune and a sign of progress.
            —*Cheri Register,* Living with Chronic Illness

Diabetes mellitus is a chronic disease that is characterized by the body's inability to regulate blood-sugar levels. A person becomes diabetic when the body can no longer properly metabolize food into energy. The two most prevalent forms of diabetes are Type 1 and Type 2. People with Type 1 diabetes, and 10 percent of the Type 2 diabetic population, require insulin injections to survive. Both types lead to secondary diseases of the nerves, eyes, kidneys, and heart. The cells that regulate sugar levels in the body fit in a thimble with room to spare, but when I was a child these cells were destroyed by my immune system, and my life was irrevocably changed by Type 1 diabetes.

I was relegated to a lifetime of trying to substitute for that tiny mass of cells by controlling the amount of sugar in my blood with insulin injections, dietary restrictions, and blood-glucose tests. It was in large part guesswork based on how food, exercise, excitement, illness, stress—indeed, all of life's variables—would affect my metabolism. And the stakes were high. Uncontrolled blood-sugar levels lead to a host of disabling complications: blindness, amputation, kidney failure, heart attacks, strokes, and premature death. Every twenty-four hours in the United States alone, diabetes causes 75 people to go blind, 80 to suffer kidney failure, and 150 to need amputations. Diabetes kills one American every three minutes; every year 2.8 million of the world's citizens die from diabetic complications. I was not alone in my childhood diagnosis. Diabetes is the leading chronic ailment among American children. Today, 135 million people worldwide have diabetes, and the numbers are rising at an alarming rate. The majority, 85 percent of those who are diagnosed with diabetes, have no prior family history of the disease. In the last forty years the incidence of diabetes has tripled, and in the next twenty years it is expected to double again. Diabetes is truly a global epidemic.

Showdown with Diabetes recounts my odyssey from the time I was ten years old. Thus, the story that follows has a course and texture familiar to anyone confronted with the relentless permanence of a chronic disease. Like a runner in a marathon, I left the starting gate believing that I could overcome the challenges of diabetes, not knowing that those challenges would become bigger, much bigger, as time wore on. As a child and then as a teen I hid my diabetes, ricocheting between denial and submission, furtively managing the multiple injections, blood-glucose tests, and doctors' appointments behind a smokescreen of bravado. But diabetes didn't slow me down. I traveled the world, snow-skied, water-skied, hiked in the Rockies, swam in the Caribbean, graduated from university and worked on Wall Street—never thinking that eye, nerve, kidney, and heart disease happened to "healthy diabetics" like me. Fifteen years into the race I felt invincible and, with no signs of secondary complications, I believed I had beaten the odds. But just as marathon runners hit a "wall" of exhaustion as their bodies' fuels are depleted, I ran headlong into a wall of secondary complications. As a young professional, I juggled my career with my secret ritual of needles and secondary diabetic complications, all the while fighting off the disruptive episodes of diabetic shock caused by low blood sugar that punctuate the lives of most diabetic people.

Within a four-year period diabetes killed the nerves below my knees, caused bleeding in the back of my eyes, the amputation of part of a toe, a skin graft, and had reduced me to needing assistance to walk. Every time something went wrong I said to myself, "If this is the worst that ever happens, I'll be fine"—but it wasn't the worst. Diabetic kidney disease set in, and every system in my body started to close down. I combed through reports of imminent cures and scientific testimonials offering "promise" and "hope." It always seemed that we were on the verge of a stunning breakthrough, but I could find no usable solutions. My career began to suffer and, living alone, unable to drive, and barely mobile due to neuropathy, the nerve disease that affects 60 percent of the diabetic population, I became a recluse. My life with diabetes became a macabre race against time as I progressed toward disability.

But here the trajectory of my story tracks in a direction largely unknown to the diabetic community; I was freed from my life of needles, restrictions, and progressive deterioration by a pancreas and kidney transplant. No more insulin injections, dietary limitations, or blood-glucose tests, yet my blood-sugar levels are normal—nondiabetic. Best of all, I am living the kind of life that I thought had passed me by. Married now, and with an expectation of a healthy future before me, I look forward to a long life with my husband. We travel widely for pleasure as well as for work, and even the simplest joys are now mine for the taking: ice cream cones on hot summer days without needing to inject insulin, long bike rides without worrying about insulin shock, and good enough vision to drive at night. I came back from the darkest of my days with diabetes to the freedoms, health, and sense of future that I had all but lost to diabetes' insidious attack.

At the end of 1996, my husband and I founded the Insulin-Free World Foundation, a nonprofit charitable organization that provides information on how advances in clinical diabetes can benefit people with diabetes now and in years to come. We have a focused objective—to act as an information exchange by compiling and redistributing information to bring science closer to people whose lives depend on it.

Today, more than seventy-five years after the first *treatments* for diabetes, we have entered the era of *cures*. Every year more than twelve hundred people are choosing to have pancreas transplants, with more than 80 percent of them being freed from their lives with diabetes. For one out of three people who live with diabetes, traditional management techniques cannot and will not prevent its deadly progress. Still, many of those in its viselike hold—joined by a medical establishment and a multi-billion-dollar maintenance industry—continue to direct their energies toward perfecting ways to live with diabetes rather than toward simpler, safer, and less expensive ways to cure it.

My objective in sharing my story is to expose diabetes so that the world will know that it is a deadly disease and that eradicating it must be a national, and international, priority. For people who are living with diabetes, I hope that my story—from diagnosis, to secondary complications, to an insulin-free life—will serve as a fire drill. Although most diabetic people will never need a pancreas transplant, it is important to know that, just in case, it is an option—and that research to improve on this solution is progressing quickly.

Part 2 of *Showdown with Diabetes* looks at the evolution of diabetes from the beginning of the twentieth century, and places the first treatments and cures within the framework of the medical advances that made them possible. For those who have witnessed or benefited from the progress made in the 1980s and 1990s, there is no question that a universal cure for diabetes is both a worthy pursuit and a very real possibility. I hope that *Showdown with Diabetes* helps to promote a community of energies—political, economic, scientific, and humanitarian—where lasting cures can quickly become a reality for all those who live with diabetes.

Part I

My Story

Prologue

Most chemists believe that the course of a chemical reaction is always predictable. But some catalytic reactions in both inorganic and organic chemistry can behave in bizarre and unruly ways.

—*Stephen Scott,* Clocks and Chaos in Chemistry

A telephone ringing nearby jarred me from a comatose sleep. The clock said three o'clock. It was teatime in London. I lay still, looking around the strange room; it was a hotel room. I was wearing my business suit. There were pages of notes beside me on the bed. Oh, no! Had I missed the meeting—and my presentation? I should have been there three hours before! I noticed two empty orange juice cans. And a candy wrapper. Had I had an insulin reaction? Yes. I remembered something. I *did* have a reaction—in the middle of my presentation! Had I embarrassed myself? What had I said? I answered the telephone wondering if it was someone from the meeting calling to tell me what had happened. It was. It was the managing director calling to congratulate me on my "spectacular performance." Spectacular? Performance? Remembering his sarcastic sense of humor, I couldn't tell what he meant by the word "performance."

"Can you meet me at the office at seven-thirty tomorrow morning?" he asked.

"Sure. I'll be there," I said and hung up. Leaning back on the pillows, I wondered out loud, "What happened at the meeting?"

The project for the large money market and foreign exchange brokerage company had been the first assignment I was given when I went to work as a researcher for an old, established executive search firm on Park Avenue in New York City. It had been my first day of work, and it hadn't started out well.

"I see here that you have diabetes." The personnel manager had said—the question was allowed in those days.

"Yes, but it isn't a problem. I'm really very lucky because I have no trouble with it."

"You'll need to fill out one more form," she said as she handed me a page with a paragraph of writing and a space for my signature and the date right below it. "It's a waiver of your rights to our life insurance policy."

"I thought life insurance is a standard benefit."

"Well, uh"—the woman cleared her throat before pressing on—"it is for everyone who's eligible, but diabetics aren't eligible for life insurance."

I paused and then asked, "And medical insurance?"

"It's standard. There's no coverage for the treatment of preexisting conditions during the first year."

I was so excited about my new job that I shrugged off the fleeting vulnerability I felt, and went to work. My first assignment had been for the financial brokerage company; they wanted us to recruit twenty-five Japanese-speaking MBAs to be trained as brokers for their offices around the world. None of the more senior researchers had wanted the assignment, preferring instead the prestige of searching for senior executives. As the new employee, I got the job, and for every executive they found I recruited ten aspiring brokers. For two weeks of every month I traveled to business schools in Europe, Asia, and throughout the United States, building relationships with placement officers and interviewing students. The travel was constant and the hours long, but I loved the work. Indeed, I had actually become quite good at it when our firm went out of business.

Right away my colleagues started to call around looking for work; my first call was to our health insurance company. I needed to know that I could have coverage while I looked for a new job. By then I had been diabetic for eighteen years, and the disease was like a monkey on my back, greedily devouring funds. No matter what, I had to feed that monkey, so medical insurance was every bit as important to me as salary. A representative at the insurance company told me I could convert my group coverage to an individual policy without being excluded for my preexisting condition, and furthermore the individual policy couldn't be terminated as long as I paid the premiums on time. The idea of securing my medical insurance, so that it could neither be terminated by the capricious whims of the market nor denied because of my preexisting condition exemption, was appealing. Without much further thought, I converted to an individual policy and struck out on my own as an independent consultant.

With medical premiums to pay and not quite sure how to get started, I called the chief executive of the brokerage firm I had been servicing and asked if I might continue the project of recruiting Japanese-speaking trainee brokers. He agreed to my proposal and so my consulting practice—headquartered out of my New York apartment—was launched.

Having no boss and no corporate structure appealed to my exaggerated need for independence, which had been fueled by my years of forced dependence on insulin, needles, and restrictions. How and when I worked were entirely my prerogative but, as my business grew, "how" became "as much as possible" and "when" was "all the time." I had always valued self-reliance and wanted to protect myself from ever being beholden to anyone or anything to help me maintain my health. The harder I worked, the more money I made, and the more independent I felt. My apartment turned into a live-in office. The telephone started ringing at 5:00 A.M. with calls from London, where it was already mid-morning. During the night, calls and faxes arrived from Asia, where the following business day was in full swing. For two weeks of every month I bounced through time zones, strange and ever-changing diets, and meetings with people who spoke languages I didn't. Diabetes became a secondary concern; with my regimen of insulin injections, glucose monitoring, and regulated meal times fitting in around my work schedule.

Diabetes had always been easy for me to hide. Few of my colleagues knew about my secret ritual of injections, blood tests, and puritanical diets. But only three years after leaving corporate America, that deception was ended by the most common secondary complication of diabetes, neuropathy, which means "nerve death." Over time, my nerves stopped sending messages to my muscles to move and, unable to move, my muscles started to atrophy. The first to go were the ones that held my feet in a right-angle position at the ends of my legs, so my feet started to "drop" slightly.

To compensate for my floppy feet I lifted my knees higher with each step, and my stride began to resemble the distinctive gait of a Tennessee walking horse. Occasionally my toes caught, and those minor stumbles sent me hurtling to the ground. My legs had skied through virgin snow in the Rockies, danced on beaches in the Caribbean, and water-skied through the waters around Bermuda, but with neuropathy, even walking was a hazardous undertaking. I started wearing only flat, flexible shoes, and for a while walking was easier. But neuropathy keeps creeping up without notice until some defining moment mocks you for what you should have felt all along.

I remember the day well—it was a Friday. I was walking with my usual distorted gait to the post office. As I waited at the corner for the light to change I noticed that several of the people who waited there too were looking, first at my feet, and then up at me. I looked down and, to my horror, saw that I was wearing only one shoe. It was like an absurd, surreal nightmare. Ashamed and flustered, I headed back home, trying to act as if nothing was wrong when I walked past the doorman into my building. He must have been as embarrassed for me as I was, because he looked away without his usual greeting. Sure enough, when I opened my apartment door I saw my other shoe sitting just inside facing out. I must have walked out of it as I was leaving.

The next morning, as I put on a pair of sneakers, I thought, *I've gone from heels to flats to lace-ups,* and I wondered when the progression would stop. In a mood of anger and hurt over my humiliation the day before, I took a taxi to Brooks Brothers on Madison Avenue to buy a cane. I knew I didn't want a standard metal, pharmacy-type cane, and I guessed that Brooks Brothers had the clientele that obliged them to carry a classier selection. I determined that if I was going to use a cane, I would make it part of my "style."

That night, in the privacy of my home, I unwrapped my new cane and looked at myself in the mirror as I leaned on it. In dizzying succession I tried on dozens of outfits—virtually everything I owned, modeling one after the other before the mirror: dresses, skirts and tops, long pants, shorts, sneakers, slippers, boots, and flat-heeled shoes. It could have been a montage of outtakes from a breezily escapist Audrey Hepburn movie except that, no matter how I looked at myself, I looked crippled. After nineteen years of hiding my diabetes, my life as an undercover diabetic was over. People would describe me as "the girl with the cane" and, quite naturally, they would wonder why I had one.

As the months passed, I felt less awkward. People looked, but rarely asked. When they did, I'd pass my cane off as something I needed temporarily to help recuperate from some made-up, nondiabetic injury or accident. I truly believed it *was* temporary, and the world didn't need to know the cause of my brief setback. For important meetings I'd leave my cane at home and, with well-honed nonchalance, compensate by leaning against walls and furniture to keep my balance.

When I received the call from the managing director of the

brokerage company's Asian subsidiaries asking me to make a presentation at their annual meeting in London, I was nervous and excited. The meeting would be a perfect opportunity to solicit more business from the Asian subsidiaries, then the fastest-growing division in the company. I was all too aware that my consulting agreement with the parent company would last only as long as there was a demand for international trainees among the regional subsidiaries. And although I knew my clients would have sympathized with my struggle with diabetes had they known of it, they were business people and would have replaced me with any one of dozens of hungry consultants on Wall Street if my productivity slipped.

My goal for my trip to London was to secure my small business's viability for the coming year by persuading the managers of the Asian offices to request more trainee brokers. But as always, to succeed I had first to succeed with the management of my diabetes. Stress always sent my blood sugar level to one of the extremes—dangerously high (hyperglycemia) or dangerously low (hypoglycemia). Either could put me in a coma. The time change between New York and London is five hours. I had flown through the night and would be speaking before this formidable group in less than four hours. Once at my hotel, I checked my blood sugar, gave myself an injection of insulin, and rested. Then I checked my blood sugar again, ate some crackers, and took a shower. At noon I was in the conference room, without my cane, confidently greeting the meeting's attendees.

We sat around a huge table, and I gave silent thanks for the luck that had us seated so I wouldn't have to worry about my balance while I gave my presentation. The meeting was called to order and, while coffee was served, the firm's managing director made opening comments. My hands were trembling imperceptibly, and I felt a cold sweat beginning to form on the back of my neck. The room started to fill with a very bright light, as though a bulb had been turned on behind my eyes. *Be calm,* I instructed myself as I rehearsed the major points of my presentation in my head. Instinctively I reached for three packets of sugar and poured them into my coffee to compensate for the glucose my body would expend from nervous energy.

All of a sudden I heard the words, ". . . and today, I've invited Deb Butterfield to speak to the international integration of our companies, and to explain how the development of multilingual brokers will support that endeavor. Deb, we're all ears." With that, the managing director sat down, and the ten top executives from Tokyo, Hong Kong, Singapore, Jakarta, Australia, and New Zealand turned to look at me.

"Thank you for the opportunity to speak here today," I began.

"Deb, would you mind going up to the podium at the end of the room so we can all see you?" the managing director asked.

"Not at all," I said with fabricated composure. *Please don't let me walk out of my shoes now,* I thought. To keep my balance, I touched the back of each chair along the side of the table as I moved toward the front of the room. Focusing intently on the ground, I lurched across the six-foot space beyond the last chair and, quickly grasping the podium, I assumed a posture of confidence.

"Is that better?" I asked.

"Yes, thank you."

"Our customers are rapidly realigning their businesses from multinational to international enterprises," I began. "Today, trading books that originate in Tokyo may be traded in London or New York. By reflecting this profile with a seamless global service, we will be in a position to compete for cross-border business. Currently . . ." A cold drop of sweat tracked slowly down my neck. The people in the room looked like they were sitting a mile away. "Ah, currently we are made up of a group of domestic companies. . . ." I kept speaking but my mind was racing. *I've got to get some sugar now. No. Keep going. You can't stop. Concentrate.* ". . . each with an independent customer base." Had I said that already? I couldn't remember. My hair was wet. My shirt was wet. My legs felt rubbery. "If an investment house is transacting business with us in Hong Kong, then it should use our . . ." *Our what?* I struggled to hang on to my main points by referring to my notes. *My sugar is too low for me to think creatively, to think at all.* After some time, perhaps twenty minutes, I heard myself summarizing the steps that I thought needed to be taken to capture cross-border brokerage activity and then—nothing.

Chapter 1

London

The worst thing that happened then, or ever in my life, was your diabetes. It was something I was completely powerless to prevent and I couldn't even take it on myself. For years and years after that moment in July, it was on my mind almost every waking moment. I'm actually thankful that the medical world painted such a rosy picture for us then, because I probably couldn't have taken it otherwise. I can only imagine what it was doing to you.

—Letter from my mother, 1990

My childhood ended and diabetes began when I was ten years old and living in London, less than a mile from the hotel where, years later, I would sit amid the orange juice cans and confusion. My family and I had moved to London after two years of living like nomads. I was born in Bermuda, the tiny island-country in the middle of the Atlantic where my father's ancestors had been among the first settlers. My mother had gone there on a two-week excursion for spring break during her junior year at university. The island was alive with calypso music and beach parties, and the men flirted with the young women who had gone to enjoy the sun and find romance.

From the first time Mom and Dad saw each other, they were inseparable, and, just four months after meeting, their whirlwind vacation romance went spinning into a wedding and an extravagant reception in Bermuda. They moved into the ancestral home next to my grandparents' house. My brother Blair, sister Lesley, and I were born while my parents were still in their twenties. But under the surface of this fairy-tale union was the mixing of two bloodlines of diabetes. Unknown to them, I had been born with the full complement of genes required to develop the disease—a ticking time bomb surrounded by a perfect world. But who would have known? Amid cheers of pride, I walked the length of the living room on my first birthday; for the next five years, people held onto lamps and breakable objects when I came into a room to protect them from my rambunctious enthusiasm.

I was five the first time I went to the mainland, during our family's summer vacation. We stayed with my great-uncle Chet and great-aunt Rache in their log cabin near Worcester, Massachusetts. Wild blueberries grew in the woods there, and I developed a passion for them. One day, armed with a bucket, I went berry picking along the wooded paths carpeted with pine needles. All morning I picked blueberries, but only half of them ever made it back to the cabin where I divided my harvest among three bowls, covered them in confectioner's sugar and took them out onto the porch to share with my great-aunt and -uncle. They were delighted and, after a few mouthfuls, asked me to go to the kitchen and get some napkins. As I walked back through the living room I saw my uncle, through the window, tossing his blueberries into the bushes. I didn't say anything when I sat back down at the table. Later, when my aunt and I took the bowls back to the kitchen to wash up, I asked her why Uncle Chet had thrown my blueberries away.

"Honey, Uncle Chet isn't allowed to eat sweet things, and he just loves you so much he didn't want to hurt your feelings by turning down your nice present."

"Why won't you let him eat sweet things?" I asked.

"Because he has diabetes," she sighed.

"He's sick?"

"Well, not really sick, because he follows a special diet and takes a medicine called insulin to keep him feeling well." Uncle Chet seemed fine so I never thought any more about it.

Four years later, when I was nine, Dad left his job at the family bank in Bermuda to take a job with a bigger bank in the Bahamas. We lived just outside Nassau on the flat, hot, and dusty main island. Nassau teemed with a desperate poverty that huddled in the shantytown "over the hill" where people had no fresh water or clothes. In flagrant contrast, the very rich lived in their private clubs with yachts and private planes. The islands were rife with political and racial unrest as Bahamians struggled for their independence from Britain. Rioting in the streets led to curfews, and burglary had reached epidemic proportions. Work permits were being taken away from non-Bahamians to create jobs for the country's citizens. For expatriates like us, there was no future in the Bahamas. With the writing on the wall, and three children and a wife to support, Dad needed a new job away from the Bahamas.

A large, international executive search firm, forever alert to changes in the currents of people's careers, approached Dad to open an office for them in London, and he grabbed the opportunity. Dad caught, quite literally, the next plane to

England to find a place for us to live. Settling quickly on an exquisite rented townhouse near Holland Park in the West End, he called for us to join him right away. We packed our things in the Bahamas, put the house up for sale, and, two days later, staggered through immigration at Heathrow airport, carrying just a few more things than we could manage. Dad picked us up in a vintage car, then drove us to the townhouse that would be our home. Blair, Lesley, and I sat in the backseat with our hair blowing in the wind as we drove along the M4 into London.

As the trees turned green with summer, I was consumed by a relentless thirst and hunger. No matter how much I drank, I was thirsty. Most days my brother, sister, and I roller-skated across the street to Holland Park and along the paths that wound through flower gardens and grassy spaces, but my body felt clumsy and lazy. More and more often Blair and Lesley had to skate in circles while I caught up. We rode to museums on the top floor of the big double-decker buses, and went to watch the guards changing shift at Buckingham Palace. Yet what I remember most about that summer was the taste of "orange squash" in little plastic containers with foil lids. Everywhere we went I wanted a drink. I'd hunt down anything wet—sodas, grapes, tea—to stop the dryness that tore at my throat and to soothe my sandpaper tongue. But nothing could stop my thirst. Ten minutes after stopping to go to the bathroom, I needed to go again. Each day I was thinner than the day before and, before long, my clothes were so baggy that Dad made extra holes in my belt to hold my jeans up.

One day the word *diabetes* lodged in my head.

"Do you think I have diabetes?" I asked Mom forthrightly.

"What? What did you say? No. Diabetes? No, of course you don't have that, sweetheart. My grandmother, your great-nanna, had diabetes. So does Great-uncle Chet. Uncle Dick does too. We would know if you had it," she said illogically and all too quickly, although the worry in her eyes reflected a greater truth that she didn't want to believe. The word *diabetes* remained silently in the air, but my unnamed disease was getting worse, and quickly. My once-rambunctious energy had been lost to the illness that reduced me to a lethargic, skin-and-bone waif. Mom knew there could be no more denying that my symptoms, our genetic predisposition, and the stress sparked by the change and uncertainty of relocating made it likely that I'd indeed developed the disease.

I will never forget that unusually hot Friday in July 1970 when she took me to see our doctor on Sloane Street. We sat in uncharacteristic silence in the sparsely furnished waiting room, needing, but not wanting, to find out what was wrong with me. No more than five minutes passed before an efficient nurse called my name. She measured and weighed me, wrote 4'10", 5 st. 2 lbs. (72 pounds) on a scrap of paper and ushered Mom and me in to see the doctor. He nodded knowingly as we explained the constant thirst and weight loss. Giving me a little plastic drinking cup, he asked me to go to the "loo" and come back with a sample of urine. The mission embarrassed me, so when I returned I surreptitiously put the cup full of urine on the edge of the sink near the door. The nurse took it and held it up to the light, then sucking in her breath she bustled off. It wasn't long before she came back and, in a kinder, more sincere tone than she had used when we arrived, asked me to let the doctor speak to my mother alone for a few minutes.

I returned to the dreary little waiting room by myself. Nervously I fingered through the magazines that were stacked neatly on the table in front of me with their worn covers. A basket of faded artificial flowers stood on the floor next to the exit, a cheerless contrast to the robust vibrancy of summer in full bloom outside. I scanned the room, searching for something that might stave off the apprehension that swelled in my belly. Looking at the chairs, I remembered the punch line of a joke Dad had told me about counting sheep. It was something to do with counting the legs and dividing by four. As I tried to fend off the nameless fear that circled around me, I counted the aluminum legs of the orange vinyl chairs and divided by four. I jumped when the door opened. Mom came over to me and I sensed that she was struggling to stay calm. Something had upset her.

"Sweetie, come with me. The doctor wants to explain the results of your tests to us." I followed her into the office.

The tension was palpable. I couldn't imagine what I'd done to make everyone so angry. The doctor was sitting behind his desk reviewing the notes he'd made in my file, perhaps wondering how to tell a ten-year-old child that she had an incurable disease; how to explain that, for the rest of her life, she must give herself multiple daily injections. How to explain to her that there was a 40 percent chance that in twenty years she would experience kidney failure. Should he tell her she had an 80 percent chance of getting eye disease? And could he explain that her life expectancy had just dropped by 30 percent?

"Debbie, the results of your tests show that you have too much sugar in your urine," he said looking at me over the top of his reading glasses to gauge my reaction.

"What difference does that make?" I asked.

"I'm afraid it means you have diabetes," he said apologetically.

I looked at Mom, and she was staring at the wall behind the doctor. Never in my life had I seen Mom cry—ever. As tears made her eyes glisten under the bright fluorescent lights, I realized that there was a lot more to diabetes than too much sugar in my urine.

"How did I catch it?" I asked trying to make some sense of what it all meant.

"Diabetes isn't contagious, anyone can get it." In those days nobody knew that diabetes is caused by the immune system attacking and destroying the insulin-producing cells in the pancreas. Neither Mom nor I said anything, so the doctor went on to explain, "Your pancreas isn't able to produce insulin anymore. Without insulin you can't convert the food you eat into energy, so the sugar builds up in your blood and spills over into your urine. The weight loss, hunger, and constant thirst that you've been experiencing are all classic symptoms of diabetes."

"Okay, so that stuff happened," I said sharply, trying to stop him from going over all the things that were wrong with me. "How can you fix it?"

"Debbie, I'm afraid diabetes can't be cured." Mom looked at me, I looked at the doctor, and he looked at Mom. My doctor, earnest, conscientious, an Everydoctor, chose, like most do, to punt: "The good news is that it's a completely manageable disease," he said buoyantly. "It'll be no problem once you get used to it." But his very word choices and explanations—"disease," "hospital," and "it can't be cured"—contradicted his platitudes. "Your mother and I think you

should come to the hospital for a little while \
your condition." I stared at Mom, hoping that sh
rect him.

"Sweetheart, we're going to be okay. We'll deal with this,"
Mom comforted. "Let's go home."

We left the doctor's office through the same doors we'd
come in just an hour earlier, but the streets of London looked
less exciting to me. From that day on I would share my body,
my experiences, and my dreams with diabetes; as I grew, so
would diabetes. Although I knew that something terrible had
just happened, fifteen years would pass before I fully appre-
ciated the severity of my diagnosis. Of course, "the future"
has little meaning to a ten-year-old child, but the permanence
of diabetes haunted my mother. *My* biggest concern was
about what would happen at the hospital the following week.
I held Mom's hand as we crossed the street to enter the
underground station. Somehow our lives had changed. We
were on a new road.

We had seen the doctor on Friday. My admission to King's
College Hospital at Denmark Hill, just south of London, was
scheduled for Monday. Over the weekend my family and I
acted as if nothing was out of the ordinary. An elephant was
in the room, but no one was talking about it. Mom masked
her feelings and kept me busy. On Saturday afternoon she
sent us children to the cinema. To this day I can't remember
which movie it was, but I do remember sneaking up the dark
aisle to the ladies' room three times. I remember stopping at
the concession stand each time for a cup of orange squash.
And I remember the bag of grapes Mom had given me to

soothe my thirst. That weekend we might just as well have been living at the turn of the century when diabetes was not understood. The treatments then were often catalysts for death. Some doctors prescribed bags of sugar, thinking they could replace the sugar that their patients lost in their urine. We thought grapes would ease my thirst and make me feel better. We didn't know that eating sugar without taking insulin could lead to the comatose death that, before the discovery of insulin, had followed in less than a year from the onset of symptoms.

Had I been diagnosed with diabetes fifty years earlier, my parents would have been carrying an emaciated child to a special hospital ward filled with the sickly sweet smell of the wasting bodies of other young diabetics in their death throes. They would have sat with me while I tried to exhale the carbon dioxide that built up in my lungs as my digestive system consumed my muscle and vital organs for energy. In those days, the only one way to slow down the process of dying was with a Draconian starvation diet known as "Allen Therapy," named for Dr. Frederick Allen, the director of the Physiatric Institute in Morristown, New Jersey, and a leading diabetologist of the time. Dr. Allen found that by virtually eliminating his diabetic patients' carbohydrate intake and urging them to consume fats to maintain their vital bodily functions, he was able to delay death. Each morsel of food was weighed and measured as if patients were monitoring their own deaths from starvation. In his book *The Discovery of Insulin*, William Bliss explains that for a twelve-year-old girl who had diabetes before insulin, "A birthday cake became a hat box covered in pink and white paper with candles on it." Allen therapy was publicly criticized for merely prolonging death, but some diabetics did endure the agony of starvation long enough to be saved by insulin.

One person to survive the diagnosis of diabetes at the beginning of the twentieth century was a fourteen-year-old named Leonard Thompson, who had fasted his way to a death-defying sixty-five pounds. His father took him to the Toronto General Hospital, but the doctors held out no hope for his recovery. As Mr. Thompson watched his son waste away, the attending physician told him about the pancreatic extract that was being developed by doctors Frederick Banting and Charles Best, who would later win the Nobel Prize for medicine for the discovery of insulin. Leonard's out-of-control high blood sugar caused his body to consume stored fat for energy. Ketone bodies (partially burned fatty acids) built up in his blood, leading to ketoacidosis. The ketoacidosis made him vomit continuously, causing dehydration. His stomach knotted in pain, and his breathing was deep and rapid. There was no doubt that Leonard would fall into a coma and die if nothing was done to intervene and, just possibly, the experimental potion the attending physician mentioned, could help. The Thompsons latched onto that shred of hope and on January 11, 1922, Leonard Thompson became the first person to be treated with insulin.

The results were astonishing. Leonard's glucose levels dropped, and his life-threatening ketoacidosis disappeared altogether. As more patients were successfully treated with insulin, it was clear that the new drug could save diabetics from a horrible and certain death. Diabetes, the once quickly fatal disease, had been transformed into a chronic and treatable condition. But for all its benefits, the discovery of insulin is a bittersweet success story because it could not then, and cannot now, replicate the body's natural regulation of glucose; in time it became clear that even with insulin, diabetes leads to a host of secondary diseases.

Not much had changed since the discovery of insulin by the time I was diagnosed in 1970, but my family and I had been spared the fear of imminent death that had been faced by Leonard Thompson and his father. There was never any question in my mind that I would be fine—diabetes, after all, could be managed with insulin. On Sunday, knowing that on Monday I would go to the hospital and get better, we piled into our old Rover car and headed to Luton, a town on the outskirts of London where Mom and Dad had been invited for the afternoon. Blair, Lesley, and I sat in the gardens and ate sandwiches while the grown-ups had a formal lunch inside the stately old mansion. I wanted a drink but I felt like I'd vomit if I had one. My legs felt like lead; I was sleepy and thirsty. Stretching out on the grass, I looked up at the elegant mansion and dreamed of one day being married at just such a place. I'd drift through the gardens in a gauzy summer dress with flowers crowning my head. Lesley would get married there too, I thought, and I'd be her maid of honor, wearing a spring hat and carrying the train of her dress in my elegantly gloved hands. As I dozed in the sun, I lost sense of time, and the afternoon seemed to blend with the night.

When Monday morning came, my parents took me in my dazed and wretched state to the big, gray hospital on Denmark Hill. Dad had arranged to take Blair and Lesley to stay with friends so that Mom could devote herself entirely to me. I smiled as I said good-bye to him, and he hugged me extra tight. As he went to leave, he said, "You can handle it, tiger." Dad always made me feel secure. He did then by downplaying the drama of diabetes and taking the burden of worry upon himself, quietly managing the logistics without ever mentioning the gnawing anxiety of paying for doctors, hospitals, and medicine—indefinitely. But I guessed at his anxiety because I had overheard his tense conversation with our medical insurance provider about preexisting conditions and how my diagnosis had come just two days before his company's new policy went into effect. And yet somehow my forever charming and creative father talked them into providing a private room for me with my own bathroom and television! I felt very important and excited, in spite of my sugar-induced confusion. Dad kissed Mom and told her he'd call us later. I waved good-bye while clicking on the television.

In short order, nurses in crisp, starched uniforms with hats that looked like the Sydney opera house began to hurry in and out of my room with lists of foods, recipes, schedules, and information about medications. They asked us lots of questions that first day. How much did I weigh? How much had I weighed six months earlier? When did my thirst start? Did anyone else in my family have diabetes? How often did I go to the bathroom? What did I eat? How much? When? I was a child, so naturally I had never paid much attention to the processes of living. I ate when I was hungry, I drank when I was thirsty, my clothes were baggy, and I didn't know how much I weighed.

My case was to be managed by Dr. David Pyke, one of Europe's leading diabetologists and world renowned for his epidemiological studies with identical twins. Dr. Pyke entered my room with an entourage of people in white coats and interrupted the interrogation. Immediately I liked this slight, friendly man with the long face, dark brown hair, and lively dark eyes. He looked like a traditional doctor with his white coat and stethoscope. He was young, too, and progressive in his approach to the role I should play in the management of my condition, introducing me to my world of diabetes with a strong emphasis on self-reliance. Dr. Pyke told me that I must learn how to make my own decisions about what to eat and how to manage insulin. "You're in the driver's seat," he said. "Doctors will be there for check-ups and crisis intervention, but you must be your own attending physician."

No more than a minute after Dr. Pyke left the room, a nurse came in with a syringe and my crash course in diabetes management began.

"What's that for?" I asked nervously.

"This is the medicine that you'll be taking twice a day from now on to control your condition," she said matter-of-factly. "It's called insulin."

"That's insulin? Nobody told me that insulin is a shot! Can't I just drink it or take a pill instead?"

"No, I'm afraid not. Insulin is a protein and the acid in your stomach would break it down before it could work." She put her hand on my shoulder and said, "Debbie, this'll get rid of your thirst and make you feel better." I clenched my teeth and squeezed my eyes closed as the nurse deftly injected the insulin into my left arm.

"That wasn't so bad," I said bravely once the danger had passed.

"Good! Because you're going to have to do the next one yourself," she said cheerfully.

"Myself? Stick a needle into myself? I can't. I can't even look!" I protested.

The nurse smiled and left us alone. I talked Mom into walking around the sterile, linoleum corridors to see what was happening on the ward. There was a woman in a green dress pushing a cart of milk and cookies. You'd have thought there was cookie rationing and that the cows had stopped producing milk the way she was carrying on with her lists of who was allowed what. I smiled and chatted pleasantly to the patients and staff we passed in the hallway, but silently I churned over and over what the nurse had said about injections and forever. Breaking my train of thought, the woman pushing the snack cart walked over and asked us to meet her back in my room. A few minutes later she came in with a basket of fruit, bread, cookies, potatoes, a kitchen scale, and a measuring cup.

"That's very nice of you. I'm starving!" I said.

"Oh dear, no," she said, sounding astonished. "You can't have a snack until your glucose level comes down. My name is Miss Wilson, and I'm a dietitian. I'm going to show you how these different foods affect your system, and I'll teach you and your mum about a diet we know of here that will help you to feel better. Let's sit down."

We sat in a row on the bed with me in the middle and Mom and the dietitian on either side. Miss Wilson explained that from then on I would eat breakfast at 7:30 in the morning, lunch at 12:30, and dinner at 6:30, with snacks midmorning, mid-afternoon, and before bed.

"This is just like Uncle Dick! Mom, he always eats dinner at exactly the same time, no matter what. Uncle Dick eats lemon on his pancakes too. He says syrup makes him sick. He can't eat cake either! Sometimes his shirts go wet with sweat and he starts shaking. Then he says candy makes him better! I have what he has, don't I? I'm going to have to live like him, aren't I?"

"You should see what they had to do before there was insulin! Back then children who had diabetes weren't allowed bread or sweets at all, and they had to eat lots of fats so they wouldn't starve to death."

"We're going to be all right," Mom said quietly, sensing my mounting anxiety.

Miss Wilson went on. "You need to learn the carbohydrate content of all the foods you eat. Every ten grams of carbohydrate is called 'one portion.' You can have four portions at each meal." She held the basket and passed a slice of bread to me, saying, "Two-thirds of this piece of bread is ten grams of carbohydrate, or one portion."

It was like arithmetic. "One piece of bread equals one and a third portions!" I said, my head beginning to twirl with numbers.

"No, not quite. A piece of bread is one and a half portions. Think about it this way. A piece of bread is fifteen grams of carbohydrates; two-thirds of that is ten grams, or one portion. The remaining five grams then is half a portion, right?"

"Oh, okay, I've got it. Sure, a piece of bread is one and a half portions, so a sandwich would have three portions of carbohydrate," I thought out loud.

I listened intently as she held up potatoes, apples, and additional slices of bread. Anyone from the outside world looking in at us sitting on that bed in the clinical white and gray room would have wondered what was so important about measuring and weighing such simple items of food. Yet, as I was to discover, calculating the carbohydrate, protein, and fat content of every meal and snack is a critical part of the diabetes equation.

Shortly after Miss Wilson left the room, another nurse came and asked Mom and me to go with her to the "lab."

"What are we going to do there?" I asked, still counting carbohydrates in my head.

"Well, I'm going to show you how to estimate how much sugar is in your body. You see, the goal is to try to keep your sugar in a normal range; insulin lowers your sugar level, and the carbohydrates and proteins that Miss Wilson was telling you about raise it."

"Really?" I asked hopefully as I roamed through the maze of information, looking for an avenue of escape.

"Yes," she said, heading off down the hallway.

"Wait a minute, I've got it! Eating will make my sugar go up and then insulin will bring it back down. I'll just do without both insulin and carbohydrates until I get better," I announced. "That'll be a whole lot easier."

She stopped and beckoned me to follow her as she said, "Don't be silly; if you don't eat you'll starve to death."

"But if I eat I'll have to take shots, right?"

"Just be thankful diabetes can be managed. Here, we're at the lab," she said as she held the door open like a sentry waiting for me to pass through.

"Pew! What's that smell?" I automatically wrinkled up my nose.

"That's urine. You'll need to collect samples of your urine throughout the day to test for sugar. You'll get used to it."

"You can't be serious!"

"Oh, yes, I'm quite serious. First you'll collect urine in a container like this one," she said holding up a plastic measuring cup. Next, with an eyedropper, you place five drops of urine into a little glass test tube, like this," she explained as she took a small sample of urine out of one of the test tubes in the wooden rack in front of her. "Then we add ten drops of water and place this pill in the mixture. It'll foam up, mind you, and can burn if it gets on your hands, so be careful. You'll need a watch with a second hand to count down sixty seconds. After one minute, hold the tube up against this chart to determine how much sugar there is in your urine. If it bubbles up orange your sugar level is too high, and if it's blue it means it's too low."

"How long will I have to do this for?"

"For the rest of your life, dear."

I felt trapped. "Everything around here is 'for the rest of my life.'" I sighed.

At 6:15 my dinner was brought in on a plastic tray. Just as I reached hungrily to lift the plastic cover off the plate, a nurse came in the door, holding a syringe, to tell me that before I ate I had to inject myself with the insulin. Mom was given an orange to practice the technique of injecting insulin, and I was given my leg. My hands started sweating. The syringe felt slippery between my fingers.

The nurse gave me instructions: "Relax your hands. Push it straight in. It hurts less if you go quickly. Count. One, two, and push. Okay, try again. One, two, and push."

I did. The needle slid into my leg. The more I concentrated on keeping my hands steady, the more they shook. The nurse went on, "Pull the plunger back to check for blood. Good, you're not in a vein. Push the plunger in. You can go faster. Push it all the way. Put your cotton swab next to the needle. Press your skin down and pull the needle out. Pull it straight so you don't bruise. Well done. Now hold your cotton swab on there to stop blood from oozing out." Mom felt faint and needed a glass of water. I felt stunned. "Now you can have your dinner, dear," the nurse said cheerfully.

I lifted the plastic cover and there, in the middle of the plate, were two egg-sized potatoes, a small piece of fish and a spoonful of green beans. For dessert I was given twelve grapes. It didn't look like dinner to me; it looked like portions of carbohydrates, proteins, and fats.

Mom stayed with me until nine that night when the nurses told her to go home and rest. "It's been a long day for you," they said, and so it had. In just one day I had learned how to stick myself with needles and how to count carbohydrates. I had heard about the peak and trough times of various types of insulin and how to test my urine for sugar. "We'll take good care of your daughter while you go home and get some sleep." Both Mom and I were exhausted, but neither one of us slept that night.

This was not the first Mom had known of adversity. She was born in a small mining town in Australia, where her father had taken a job as a geologist after receiving his doctorate in geology from Yale University. When she was nine she moved to Zacatecas, Mexico, where Grandad had accepted an offer to work with an American mining company. Life in mining towns was violent. Mom can still picture the machine guns set up along their driveway, and the night that her best friend's father was stabbed to death during a union dispute. Nonetheless, Mom had seen the romance and adventure in her life and had never lost her natural optimism. She believed that every story, no matter how gloomy or uncertain, should have a happy ending. Much later, Mom told me about the night she left me at the hospital, about how she had been inconsolable. She cried and railed against the enemy she couldn't see, the enemy that had slipped past her protective barriers and now lived in her child. She would have done anything to drain the diabetes from my body and take it on herself. That night she vowed she would find a way to free me of diabetes.

After Mom left for the night, tears of exhaustion and unspent emotion streamed down my face. A sense of panic betrayed the smiles I had worn all day. I wanted to run away from that gray, antiseptic-smelling place and from the disease I didn't want, as if I could leave it there along with my hospital gown. There was an enemy in my body and I was in a strange place with a disease I didn't understand. The nurses spoke with English accents, and their words were foreign: Clinitest, insulin, ketones, hypoglycemia. I tried to look inside myself for answers, but there weren't any. I was ten years old, alone with my diabetes, and somehow I knew that I always would be.

The phone rang beside my bed. It was Dad calling from the south coast, just as he had promised. He told me jokes to make me laugh, as he always could. Dad was the most exciting person in the world to me. I used to love going to the airport in Bermuda to welcome him when he came home from his business trips. Dad was always easy to pick out of the crowd of passengers because he'd be the one carrying some funny souvenir he'd picked up along the way for us. Talking to Dad, and being in the hospital with diabetes, made me remember my birthday two years earlier, and the three-foot-tall piñata he'd brought back from South America for me.

To a child growing up in the tropics where it never snows,

a piñata in the form of a snowman, down to its big orange nose and black felt hat, creates its own excitement. But Mom decided also to make it the theme of my birthday party. She baked a fabulous snowman-shaped cake, covered it with white icing and coconut flakes, made a mouth out of licorice, and, of course, the nose was a carrot. My guests and I, all dressed up in our party clothes, wore cheerful paper hats as we sat around the big table Mom had adorned with little baskets of jellybeans and party favors. We ate barbecued hot dogs and hamburgers, and cheered when Mom and Dad walked out with my beautiful snowman cake all ablaze with candles. Everyone sang "Happy Birthday" to me. My face muscles ached from smiling as I blew out the eight little flames that flickered on the striped green and yellow candles. Mom cut each of us a big wedge of the moist, yellow snowman cake with its creamy icing that stuck the layers together; but she gave Tony, one of the little boys who lived farther around the harbor, a bowl of fruit salad. I looked quizzically at Mom and she whispered, "Cake makes Tony sick." Everyone ate with gusto, right down to the last exquisite indulgence of sucking the icing from our fingers—that is, everyone except Tony. He counted each bite of fruit he ate and studiously left the last four grapes.

After lunch we played games: pin the tail on the donkey, Simon says, and musical chairs. All of this led up to the crescendo, breaking open the snowman piñata that Dad had attached to a tree behind the house. Because I was the birthday girl I went first. As I swung wildly in the air, my friends clamored, "My turn, my turn." When my cousin Mark broke the snowman wide open, everyone shrieked with delight and dove for the candies and trinkets lying like treasure at our feet. But not Tony; he just stood on the side watching. I called to him to join us, not to be shy, but he just smiled and shook his head. Another of my friends bellowed, "Tony sticks himself with needles so he can't eat candy or have presents," and someone else chimed in, "When he cheats, he can't eat sweets." Tony looked sad and angry all at once. As I sat in King's College Hospital I finally understood that look I had seen in Tony's eyes.

Mom, I knew, would always worry about my diabetes and would try too hard to manage my problem for me. Blair and Lesley would help me to hide my "secret" from the world; and Dad of course would try even harder to fill my days with fun. But when all was said and done, only I could live the diabetic life I'd inherited.

The doctors had said I'd have no trouble with diabetes once I was more familiar with it, and I too was convinced that once I got used to the insulin injections all would be fine. I knew I was lucky not to have cancer or epilepsy, and I felt ashamed for the "Why me?" I wanted to scream at the world. Yet, with the resilience of a marathoner at the start of a race, my spirits bounced back and, by the next morning, I felt much better. I was less thirsty, and my head felt clearer. For the first morning in a long time I jumped out of bed without feeling like I wanted to sleep all day. All in all, I felt up to the challenge of diabetes and started asking about how soon I could go home.

Some years later, I came across a nurse's reminiscences of the 1920s scene as young diabetic patients like myself waited for their doctor, Dr. Allen, to arrive with some of the first bottles of the then newly discovered insulin. It brought home to me what a truly valuable discovery insulin was:

The mere illusion of new hope cajoled patient after patient into new life. Diabetics who had not been out of bed for weeks began to trail weakly about, clinging to walls and furniture. Big stomachs, skin-and-bone necks, skull-like faces, feeble movements, all ages, both sexes—they looked like an old Flemish painter's depiction of a resurrection after famine. It was a resurrection, a crawling stirring, as of some vague springtime. . . . My office opened on the big center hallways. I could see them drifting in, silent as the bloated ghosts they looked like. Even to look at one another would have painfully betrayed some of the intolerable hope that had brought them. So they just sat and waited, eyes on the ground.

It was growing dark outside. Nobody had yet seen Doctor Allen. . . . We all heard his step coming along the covered walk, past the entrance to the main hallways. His wife was with him, her quick tapping pace making a queer rhythm with his. The patients' silence concentrated on that sound. When he appeared through the open doorway, he caught the full beseeching of a hundred pairs of eyes. It stopped him dead. Even now I am sure it was minutes before he spoke to them, his voice curiously mingling concern for his patients with an excitement that he tried his best not to betray.

"I think," he said, "I think we have something for you."

Insulin was not a cure, but it *had* saved my life. Within a week I was back home and full of energy. My laughter and sense of excitement returned and I felt better than I had in months. My thirst disappeared, and flesh and muscle began again to fill out my gaunt, thin frame; but I had changed, and so had my family. Blair and Lesley asked me about the hospital and about taking injections. Rather than sharing the jumbled, scared thoughts on the tip of my tongue, I answered them with a bravado I didn't feel—a public posture regarding my diabetes that would become as familiar to me as the daily insulin that sustained me. I was, and would remain, embarrassed by diabetes, by testing my urine, by giving myself injections, and, like Tony, by not being allowed candy and cakes.

I had felt scared by the shaky, sweaty headachy episodes of disorientation I had experienced that summer when my sugar levels dropped too low. But instead of sharing this with Blair and Lesley, my two closest allies, I told them, "If I take care of myself, I'll live a normal and healthy life." I steered the conversation away from me and told them about the people I had met in the hospital. How could I explain my visit to the lab with the little glass tubes of urine lining the counter? How could I explain the diet to them when I still wasn't sure I understood it myself? And so I retreated behind a wall of smiles, echoing Mom's words of comfort—*Everything will be all right*—and I willed myself to believe that it would.

Chapter 2

School Years

We are the carriers of lives and legends—who knows the unseen frescoes on the private walls of the skull.
　　　　　　　　—William Goyen, The House of Breath

F	our weeks after completing my course on diabetes man-
	agement at King's College Hospital I left home to go to
	Cobham Hall, a stately boarding school in the country-
side of Kent. The school, once the home of an English noble-
man named Lord Darnley, was an age-softened brick building
with leaded glass windows and imposing stone hallways. It had
served as a field hospital during the War of the Roses. The
tramping of many armored men and slippered noble folk had
worn the majestic, cold stone stairways to a smooth, soft finish.
Cobham Hall was a five-minute walk along an earthen country
lane from a hamlet that was no more than a church, a post office,
a tobacconist's, a tea shop, and a small collection of cottages.

Earlier in the summer, before that defining moment in July when I'd been diagnosed with diabetes, a list of clothing and sundries required for attendance at the school had arrived in the mail. We were instructed to make our purchases of the listed articles at the John Lewis department store and to sew name tags into each item. Mom, Lesley, and I had gone to the store on Oxford Street on one of the big, red double-decker buses that had seemed so unusual to us when we first moved to London. How we laughed when Mom read off the items I'd be needing from the list of required clothing: "White plimsols, a sponge bag, three frocks, a boater, two pairs of bloomers, seven pairs of knickers . . ."

"Stop! Stop! Two pairs of blooming what?" I asked laughing. "Three flocks of what? A boat? I think I'm going to like this school!"

Cobham was the third new school I had attended in less than two years. I'd always enjoyed meeting people and making new friends, but this time my enthusiasm was dampened by my apprehension about managing diabetes in a strange place, and by knowing that I had to do it all by myself. My classmates included titled nobility, foreign royalty, and daughters of members of Parliament, but the school emphasized our similarities by standardizing the blue-and-white checked skirts, white cotton shirts, blue overcoats, and oatmeal-colored socks that we wore. What we did and what we learned were predestined—being different, or spontaneous, wasn't a virtue. The food chain started with the headmistress and teachers at the top, then senior girls and prefects, on down to the girls my age, who had no say whatsoever in the scheduling of our days. The very youngest girls slept in two large dormitories, each with fourteen beds. Because I was in the second year, I was assigned to a smaller room with eight beds. The room was on the top floor at the end of a long, dark hallway lined with wooden wardrobes. At the foot of each of the metal-frame beds that lined the walls was a wooden chair. We each had a wooden dresser with three small drawers, and a third of one of the wardrobes in the hallway outside, to store our clothes.

The week before the start of school, my parents had received a letter from the school's physician to say that my syringe and insulin would need to be kept under lock and key in the dispensary, at all times. After leaving my suitcase on a bed in the corner of the room, we went to find the small room, no bigger than a large closet, where the school nurse tended to the minor colds and calamities of her charges. An old wooden table with a Formica top and metal legs stood next to the door, and a friendly-looking nurse wearing a white uniform and starched hat was making notes in a big book. Dad waited in the hallway while Mom and I went to talk to her; as we approached I clung to the blue canvas bag holding my supply of insulin, dozens of needles, and a glass syringe in its sterilizing kit.

"Hello. I'm Sara Butterfield and this is my daughter Deborah," Mom said boldly.

"Welcome to Cobham, Debbie. Mrs. Butterfield, I received your letter explaining your daughter's illness."

"I'm not ill," I said quickly as I tried to familiarize myself with the strange little room where I would take care of my diabetes. A cupboard with glass doors hung on one of the walls and held bottles of aspirin, cough syrup, Band-Aids, and other small emergency equipment. Beneath the cupboard was a sink embedded in a white counter. "Where should I keep my insulin and syringe?" I asked.

"Oh, just put them on the counter," the nurse smiled. "Dispensary is open for half an hour before breakfast and dinner, so you must always stop here for your insulin injection on your way to the dining room. Do you have a letter for me from your doctor to explain your insulin doses?"

"Deborah will explain everything you need to know about her diabetes. She knows what to eat and how much insulin to take; she will always make her own decisions about those things," Mom interjected quietly, but firmly.

"My diabetes is really no problem. You needn't worry about me," I said trying to ease the tension.

Mom went on, explaining that she wanted to be called immediately when, not if, things went wrong. In the short time since leaving the hospital, we had already learned how unpredictably my blood sugar could swing from high to dangerously low.

"You'll be the first to know," the nurse said comfortingly.

"Nothing's going to go wrong," I reassured them. "I'll be fine."

The nurse put her hand gently on my shoulder as she stopped an older girl in the hallway and asked her to take us to join the other students for tea. Several tables had been set up in the cavernous, wood-paneled dining hall, with pots of tea, milk, sugar, and little sandwiches. I was full of the nerves and excitement of being the new girl; and my hands trembled and my palms felt clammy. Glancing at my watch I saw it was already 4:00, an hour after I should have had my snack. I realized that my shaking hands and sweaty palms were due not to nerves but to hypoglycemia. I needed some carbohydrates, and soon. I whispered in Mom's ear that I'd left my glucose tablets in my room and automatically she reached for a bowl of sugar and spooned some into a cup of milk for me. I drank it quickly and then filled the cup again and drank that too. The girl who had escorted us downstairs watched me curiously and asked politely, "Do you not like tea?"

"Oh yes, really I do! But I was a little too hot for tea today," I said awkwardly, realizing right away that my response was inconsistent with the chill in the draughty old dining room on that damp September day. I was saved from further explanation by the announcement that blared over the public-address system that it was time for our families to leave. I smiled through tears as I walked Mom and Dad to the front door. "I'll write soon," I said flatly as I kissed them good-bye and went back to my room to meet my new roommates.

A matron stopped me at the door and told me to unpack my suitcase and line up my belongings on my bed in the order that they appeared on the clothing list. Before long, she came in to inspect the name tags on each item, right down to the last sock and handkerchief. Checking them off against the list, she said that I'd be responsible for anything that was missing at the end of the term. Without taking a breath, she launched into a litany of rules and regulations: when I could wash my hair; when to write to my parents; what to wear; when to eat; what to eat; when to sleep; and when to study. As she spoke I scrambled to fit her rules into the stream of diabetic rules running through my head: when to eat; what to eat; when to exercise; how much insulin to take; and when to test my urine for sugar. Teatime would be at 4:20 every day, but my diabetes needed a snack at 3:00. Tea was jelly donuts, but my diabetes needed fruit or plain cookies. Chapel would be on Sunday mornings; of course, there was to be no eating in church. Church or not, my diabetes needed a snack in the middle of the morning.

There were small metal lockers stacked five deep and running the length of the "Blue Corridor," named for the eerie blue glow from the dim lights at night. Each of us was assigned a locker where we kept valuables and were allowed to keep candy, but only candy. We were expressly forbidden to keep any other type of food, yet I had to have crackers and plain cookies for snacks when my insulin was at its peak reaction time. Every three weeks when I went home, Mom supplied me with a stock of cookies, and I knew exactly how many equaled "one portion." Mom also made sure to send me back with at least a dozen packets of Dextrosol. Dextrosol was fast-acting glucose tablets that I took to recover from hypoglycemia. They'd become such a familiar part of our life at home that Blair developed a song about them. To the Carole King song *"You've Got A Friend,"* he'd bellow tunelessly:

> *You just call Dextrosol*
> *And you know wherever I am*
> *I'll come running*
> *To save you again.*

Unlike the other girls' lockers, mine held no comforting chocolates or gummy bears. It was more medicine chest than treasure chest. In the middle of the morning and in the afternoon I'd go there only to count and consume carbohydrates to stop my blood sugar from crashing between meals. Every morning I went to my locker and put exactly four cookies in each of two plastic bags, breaking them into small pieces so I could suck them until they slid down my throat without being noticed. Occasionally the matrons checked our lockers for contraband and, inevitably, they'd confiscate my supplies. I felt humiliated having to beg to get them back, as if I was a criminal for having them in the first place. My explanations invariably aroused their pity, as well as my anger at being so dependent on the cookies—and insulin.

Knowing what dose of insulin to take was not a precise science then, and it isn't now. In those days, with only urine testing as a guide, it was like playing darts while wearing a blindfold. But I believed that diabetes *could* be managed, and was frustrated by my inability to control it. At the same time as I wrestled with controlling my diabetes, I was trying to protect my identity as "just one of the gang." What would my new friends think if they knew I tested my urine for sugar by mixing it with acid tablets in a test tube? What would they think of my boiling a syringe to sterilize it and inject myself with insulin twice a day? How would they react when I started sweating and shaking and needed to eat candy? Or when my vision blurred and I felt confused because my blood sugar was too high or too low? Diabetes was part of me, and yet diabetes didn't fit in. If the other girls thought these unnatural things I did were "weird," they'd laugh at me, tease me, or worse still, exclude me.

During those formative years when so much of my sense of self was a reflection of what others thought of me, I avoided people's reactions to my diabetes by living undercover, behind the wall of silence and smiles I had established shortly after my diagnosis. Nondiabetic people have asked me why I was so secretive about my diabetes. Perhaps I can explain it like this. Think back to when you were in junior high. How would you have felt if you were told in driver's ed. that you couldn't get a license without a doctor's certificate? What would you have said if blood seeped through your shirt from injecting insulin and someone asked you what it was? Would you have been angry if you were banned from a sports team because you were diabetic? How would you have felt if people told you what you should and shouldn't eat? What would you have done if you were in the middle of an exam and started sweating profusely and couldn't remember why you were there? How would you have felt if word got out that you tested your urine for glucose? Diabetes is a master at creating moments like these. Cobham Hall was my whole world. My friends there were my family. I lived there. I needed to fit in.

My happiest moments were when I was playing on the school netball, rounders, and swim teams. Every two weeks or so we had a game away and could escape the restrictive confines of the boarding school property for an afternoon. Swim team was my favorite. The feel of the soothing water against my skin carried me back in time to my fairy-tale Bermuda childhood—my life before diabetes. The team practiced during lunch hours so our meal was delayed until practice was over. My morning insulin peaked at lunchtime so the delay, in addition to the exercise that would burn up sugar, was a problem. The thing I feared most about diabetes was hypoglycemia: the feeling of slipping beyond conscious control; scrambling for thoughts; soaking in cold sweat; fumbling for sugar; muscles locking. And then nothing. Hypoglycemia can lead to coma and death, and it is the most swiftly fatal of all of the complications of diabetes. On the days the swim team met, I'd adjust my morning insulin and snack to compensate as well as I could for the late lunch and extra exercise. My anxiety about hypoglycemia's interfering with my performance was most pronounced at the beginning of each term during the two weeks leading up to try-outs. I'd test my urine and take insulin with devout attention to each minor physical and emotional variance. Urine testing was inaccurate and it was hard to know whether or not my efforts actually improved my overall blood-sugar levels, but psychologically "being in control" helped me to fight my fear of hypoglycemia.

At the beginning of my third year, I was standing at the side of the pool waiting for my turn when my hands started to tremble ever so slightly. Sweat crept down my back and broke out on my forehead. The pool and my friends looked small and distant, as if I was looking at them through the wrong end of a telescope. When my name was called, I moved with heavy legs to the edge of the pool. When the starting gun sounded, I dove in. I knew I should have stopped first to eat some Dextrosol tablets but instead I said to myself, *Just one more minute. Swim team is more important.* I swam as fast as I could and saved precious nanoseconds by not taking breaths as I churned through the water. Reaching out to take a stroke, my hand came crashing down on the cement of the pool's edge. *That must be my best time ever*, I thought as I pulled myself out of the pool. But I could hear my friends laughing and calling, "Hey idiot, you're supposed to swim the *length* of the pool, not the width!" My legs gave way as I tried to stand, and I fell to the ground vomiting and shaking. My head felt like it was in a vise. The lifeguard called the nurse, but I didn't get enough sugar fast enough to stop me from passing out on the way to the infirmary. When I woke up, my hand was wrapped in bandages and the nurse was beside me holding a package of Dextrosol.

"Did they throw me off the team?" I asked anxiously.

"No, but *I've* taken you off and declared you medically unfit," she said angrily. "If you had eaten lunch on time and not been down at that pool swimming, you wouldn't be lying here with a broken thumb—you should've known better."

I closed my eyes, vowing that I wouldn't let her or anyone else set priorities for my health and my life. Those who knew I had diabetes treated me differently by being overly protective or by lowering their expectations of me. Like the school nurse, some became instant police, passing disapproving judgments on what I ate or how I managed my time or activities. The only way I knew how to stop people from encroaching was to hide my diabetes. The nurse called Mom and, without a moment's hesitation, she drove an hour and a half along the country lanes through the fields of Kent to be by my side. She took me home and for the next three days and nights, she brought me fluids, insulin, and crackers. Every four hours, day and night, she tested my urine for sugar, and when the acid that bubbled to the top of the test tube turned green, she took me back to Cobham.

I had learned a great deal about diabetes in a few short years, and as I did I moved further away from the rosy picture that had been painted at the outset. Diabetes in the real world was substantially different from what it had been in the controlled environs of the hospital at Denmark Hill where I had first learned about the balance of insulin, food, and exercise. Holidays, exams, travel, excitement, infection, colds, anxiety—these everyday events derailed my ability to control diabetes, just as diabetes itself was beginning to derail my life. I'd lost my place on the swim team because I had mis-managed diabetes, not because I couldn't swim fast enough. To fulfill my ambitions I had first to control diabetes, and to do that I had to factor diabetes into all my decisions. Never-theless, Mom still clung to the cheery "everything will be fine" view that had helped her to cope when I was diagnosed. I think she believed that through sheer will and optimism she could keep me healthy forever. In a June 1974 letter to my grandparents at the end of my fourth year of school in Eng-land (equivalent to sophomore year in high school), she wrote:

Deborah has finished her exams as of yesterday, although the hard ones were finished last week. She went on an out-ing to Cambridge on Tuesday, a day trip on the hovercraft to France (Boulogne) on Wednesday, and to the tennis at Wimbledon on Thursday, so she's having a very exciting last two weeks of school.

Beneath the veneer, the truth was somewhat different. I recall a week with sky-high blood sugars, of sitting on buses, of worry, of tremendous thirst, and of feeling like my bladder would explode. I remember asking the bus dri-ver to stop three times in two hours for a rest room, explaining it away as carsickness. I have memories of pass-ing out on the hovercraft because lunch was an hour late, of getting back to school after the infirmary had closed and breaking in to get my insulin. All in all, diabetes had undermined a week of enormously privileged opportu-nity—yet I too talked about those exciting last two weeks of school as they should have been. I talked about how I'd spoken French in France, the strawberries I'd eaten at Wimbledon, and the warm, fresh Cornish pastries I'd devoured while boating on the "backs" of Cambridge, the river that flows through the fields behind Cambridge University. Like Mom, I talked about the world as I wanted it to be, not as it was. My undercover life with diabetes had become so remote from my public persona that it no longer penetrated the surface. After "lights out," I'd lie looking at the ceiling and thinking about what it would be like after school was over. I dreamed of having a large family where we'd talk about everything that mattered and lots of things that didn't. There would be laughter and tears and we'd have picnics, hold hands, and watch the sun go down. When I pictured my future, there was no diabetes.

Chapter 3

A Healthy Diabetic

Ignorance is a necessary condition for many excellent things. The childish joy of seeing what Santa Claus has brought for Christmas is a species of joy that must soon be extinguished in each child by the loss of ignorance.

—*Daniel C. Dennett,* Darwin's Dangerous Idea

When I was fifteen my parents divorced, and I moved to the United States with my mother. Again I went to boarding school, this time to Chatham Hall in southern Virginia where my sister Lesley had spent her senior year. I'd only ever been to the States on vacation and, despite the sadness I felt at the end of my parents' marriage, I was thrilled by the brashness of America and by the great adventure of moving there. I adapted quickly to the new vernacular and way of life. "Chips" became "french fries," and I traded in my English trousers and plimsols for blue jeans and sneakers.

The people in the small town just down the road from the

red brick buildings and white-steepled church of Chatham Hall were gentle, God-fearing folk with a deep commitment to family. Music of all kinds—bluegrass, spiritual, folk—was an important part of their lives. The girls at school who'd grown up in Virginia would pick up guitars and sing as easily as the rest of us would turn on the radio. Altogether, Chatham Hall should have been a safe place to be during those years when the forces of adolescence sparked teenage rebellion, but being a teenager in a diabetic body was far from safe.

From the day I was diagnosed, the medical profession had hidden the progressive nature of diabetes. "You can live a normal healthy life," they said. "Diabetes is controllable." "With your attitude, it'll be no problem." My upbeat and hopeful family reminded me that my Uncle Dick, great-uncle Chet, and great-grandmother had all been "healthy diabetics." Only Mom's cousin Mac had trouble, but everyone said it was because "he didn't take care of himself." So I took care of myself. My daily schedule of insulin injections and of counting carbohydrates and proteins was as much a part of my routine as brushing my teeth.

Few people knew about that part of me I hated. My diabetes didn't show, and most of the time it didn't affect how well I felt. Because I wasn't ill, and didn't look sick, I felt an asymmetry between my health and having a chronic disease. Like my relatives before me, I was a "healthy diabetic," a contradiction in terms like a "minor disaster," or "bad health." Having diabetes was tantamount to living in a box; the penalties for stepping outside the box were harsh. Beyond the acute complications of hypoglycemia and ketoacidosis, each elevated blood-sugar level was another step toward the long-term irreversible complications that can lead to blindness, kidney failure, amputations, and heart disease. Most of the time I managed to manipulate my schedule to accommodate diabetes, but I engaged in a secretive and willful struggle between staying in my box and indulging in the life that beckoned outside. Somewhere in that conflict I was trying to find the right balance between being limited by my health and deluding myself that diabetes was "no problem."

The introduction of insulin was a double-edged sword. Without question insulin made it possible to live with a disease that before had promised only death. But insulin led society to believe that diabetes is no more than a chronic and manageable condition; because it was no longer fatal, the focus of diabetes research shifted away from finding cures to finding ways to improve management. The diabetic population became a captive customer base and so, logically, diabetes quickly became a thriving commercial industry. Even the small drug store in Chatham sold disposable syringes of several sizes and gauges; beef and pork insulin of different durations; Tes-Tape; Clinitest; alcohol swabs; carrying cases for paraphernalia; and myriad glucose products. The local bookstore carried shelves of cookbooks with diabetes "exchange" lists and books on living well with diabetes. Nonprofit organizations and associations had been established to support and educate the large diabetic population. The grocer carried a wide range of sugar-free goods. Yet no combination of these products and services could actually perfect glucose control. Smaller needles, disposable syringes, and sugar-free food and drinks provided no more, and no less, than ways to simplify the process of trying. The next significant advance in diabetes management, blood-glucose monitors, was made in 1980, over half a century after the discovery of insulin.

Dr. Michael Miller met the venture capitalist Ted Doan at a cocktail party. Miller shared with Doan his belief that urine testing was inconvenient and, more importantly, an inaccurate way for diabetics to try to determine how much insulin or food they needed at any given time. Dr. Miller explained that monitoring glucose in the blood would show current glucose levels—at that moment—whereas the urine testing we had relied on was, at best, a delayed estimate of how much excess sugar had spilled into the urine from the blood during the previous few hours. Dr. Miller reasoned that testing sugar in the blood could give diabetics vital information to calculate insulin doses and dietary allowances more accurately. Dr. Miller convinced Mr. Doan, and together they developed a blood-glucose monitor.

News about blood-glucose monitors appeared in pharmacy ads and diabetes magazines everywhere. At first the monitors and test strips cost hundreds of dollars; insurance would not pay for them. They were cumbersome, too. Testing was complicated and took five minutes, but for the first time it was possible for diabetics to know exactly how much sugar was in their bloodstream any time of day or night. I was so excited about the wonderful new machines that I raced right out and bought one, along with packets of lancets and test strips. I fully believed that it would be my ticket to controlling diabetes. I designated a pocket in my backpack for my new diagnostic toy and carried it everywhere. After a few months I both loved and hated my monitor. On the one hand, being able to detect swings in my blood-sugar level before it reached extreme highs or lows made me feel less vulnerable to being caught off guard by hypoglycemia. On the other hand, the cold, unforgiving numbers that flashed across the screen often defied logic, having little to do with the amount of effort I had put into managing my diabetes. Sometimes, with little work at all, they would hover in the normal range for weeks; sometimes, despite my most dedicated attempts, they bounced from high to low and back again. The harsh and despotic justice pushed me to rages of frustration. My monitor displayed its last incomprehensible test result in one such rage because I threw it out of a third-floor window.

Squeezed between peer pressure and the dispassionate authority of diabetes, my teenage years were lived in conflict between complying with my diabetic regime and making choices in spite of it. My friends exercised their adolescent rebellion by drinking alcohol or taking drugs, but I'd go to Häagen-Dazs for a milkshake or stop at Dunkin' Donuts; then I'd take insulin to try to counteract the overload of glucose. My friends were proud of their rebellion, but I was consumed by a sense of failure. When my glucose levels were too high or too low I was angry, not at diabetes, but with myself. My self-esteem dissolved in the face of what I perceived to be my lack of will. From a high-spirited, life-is-a-blast child of the tropics, I had become a compromising, isolated teenager hiding behind a mask of easy laughter and a wide smile.

By my senior year of high school, I'd been diabetic for almost seven years and had started to form a more potent understanding of my disease. I was all too aware that controlling blood-sugar levels isn't a simple algorithm of food, insulin, and exercise. The multifaceted equation includes stress, excitement, delayed meals, meals in restaurants, travel, infections, colds, unscheduled activities, and, of course, adolescence. Intellectually I knew elevated blood-sugar levels could have disabling consequences, but as with fires and natural disasters, the possibility lived in that part of my psyche that says to people, "Those things happen to others, not to me."

The challenge of being a diabetic child had been to coordinate the rules of diabetes with the school rules. But as a sixteen-year-old, I started questioning those very tenets and felt cheated by the restraints of diabetes that barred me from the random pleasures of adolescence. The evolution from childhood to adulthood is a time of profound change and diverse experience, neither of which are conducive to stable diabetic control. I lost faith in doctors who made the overly simplistic and condemning assertion that diabetes could be controlled simply by being "compliant" with a prescribed regimen of insulin injections, blood-sugar tests, and diet. When the novelty of glucose monitors had worn off, it was clear that no amount of monitoring and no number of insulin injections could replicate the thermostatic speed and accuracy of a normally functioning pancreas.

As the years went by, I realized that the doctors' platitudes had been no more than evasive phrases of comfort, perhaps because they had believed that the truth about diabetes, especially the absence of solutions, was not a child's domain. The half-truths, like those about Santa Claus, had been compassionately misleading and had indeed allowed me the unquestioning optimism of childhood. From my vantage point then, diabetes was no more than an inconvenient condition that needed to be monitored.

Discovering the whole truth about diabetes reminds me of

that old story about the blind men on safari who happen across an elephant. Each of them holds onto the beast and describes what he has caught. "I've caught a long snakelike beast" screams the one holding the tail. "Oh my," says the man hugging the elephant's leg, "I have a wrinkly, leathery animal that feels like a tree trunk." A man hanging onto the elephant's ear pipes up, "Oh no, it's a flat, oval, fuzzy one!" Of course they are all right, but without the full picture none of them could identify the elephant. And so it is with diabetes. Diabetes is a complex disease that can lead to a host of other diseases of the eyes, nerves, kidneys and heart. Different people develop diabetes at different ages and not all diabetics suffer from the same secondary complications over the same period of time, or to the same degree.

The picture of diabetics living active, seemingly normal lives, with no apparent manifestations of their disease, is only part of the "elephant." I was at risk of being trampled by the parts I could not see. Experience had taught me that the mantra "Diabetes is compatible with a healthy and happy life-style" wasn't the whole truth. Diabetes doesn't fit into a life-style—it dictates it. And even the most rigorous attempts to control diabetes offer no guarantees of health. Diabetes is more than just taking insulin. Insulin injections have become a symbol, an expression of the disease, but the disease itself transcends the physical acts required to try to control it.

Sometime during my adolescence I realized I had to start making choices, as a diabetic, about whether or not to have the adventures that most people take for granted as formative experiences in developing their personality and their identity. I needed to decide when to avoid those opportunities and when to enter environments of excessive or undue risk to

cross a frontier in my own understanding of life beyond diabetes. It was just such a decision I made when, after graduat-
ing from high school, I signed on as a crew member on a
forty-five-foot yacht that needed to be delivered from
Bermuda to St. Barth's to be chartered out for the winter. I
had been raised on my father's story of the winter of 1955,
when he joined a crew in England to sail home to Bermuda.
Sailboats had been more familiar to Dad than cars. He had
learned celestial navigation about the time he had learned to
read, so the idea of sailing a boat to Bermuda was no more
than a youthful adventure. It had been fine weather as the
White Cliffs of Dover receded on the horizon, but out in the
Atlantic, their small sailboat was driven off course by a water-
spout, a tornado on the ocean. Their navigation equipment
was destroyed in the storm. They were adrift for six weeks
with only the rainwater they could catch to drink, and days
without food, before they washed up on the shores of
Antigua. Dad said he had left England as a boy and arrived in
Bermuda a man. I had always admired and tried to emulate
Dad's explosive enthusiasm for life and, although I didn't
want to get lost at sea, I wanted to go on the trip to St.
Barth's. I wanted to understand my strengths and fears from
being at sea with just a boat, a crew, and the forces of nature.

St. Barth's is an island in the southern Caribbean. We
would have a straight seven-day, seven-night sail through the
Bermuda triangle. Our shifts were four hours on and four
hours off—day and night. Our second night out, I was on
the midnight to 4:00 A.M. shift with my watch partner when
we hit a squall. For two hours, the two of us took turns
pulling ourselves to the foredeck to reef the sails, free sheets,
and check hatches. All the while, we were hooked to the

boat's railing with lifelines in case we were washed overboard. Back in the cockpit we strained against the wheel to keep the boat on course as waves crashed over the deck and the boat slammed into the troughs between waves. As the storm intensified we called all hands on deck. The seven of us worked through that storm until the middle of the next day. When we sailed out of the far side of the storm, we were exhausted and exhilarated, with a sense of having survived a very big and stormy ocean in a very small boat. I treasured that experience of staring into danger with my peers, and knowing that we were all taking the same risk. When we arrived in St. Barth's, I hitchhiked to the airport and flew back to my family's home in Bermuda to pack my things and head off to university.

Three days later, I was registering for classes for my first semester at the University of Colorado in Boulder. Once again, I chose not to tell my university friends about my diabetes. I wanted to fit in by doing the same things my college friends did: occasionally staying up all night, skipping a meal, studying until very late, or saving time in the morning by eating breakfast before going to sleep. But the microvascular and neurologic changes taking place in my body were very different from the nondiabetic resilience of theirs.

As a sophomore I volunteered at the university's theater, where I helped to build stage sets, find props, and make costumes. The joy and energy I found there intoxicated me. When the academic year was over I auditioned for, and was accepted to, the American Academy of Dramatic Arts in New York City. New York was expensive, so I took two part-time jobs, one a weeknight position as a hostess at a small East Side restaurant, and the other as a weekend tour guide at South Street Seaport. I attended class from 8:00 A.M. to 4:00 P.M., then I'd catch a bus uptown where I'd work at the restaurant until eleven. On weekends I gave tours of the great ships—the large sailing vessel *Peking,* and the lightship *Ambrose.* It was a frenetic time.

Acting school taught me to express myself through the characters on the page, and it gave me a risk-free outlet for much of the frustration and anger I harbored. It also taught me to seek perfection in both the look and the performance of my body. I measured my discipline by how well I managed my diabetes. My regimen went beyond mere good control; a secret pride grew inside me for my puritanical will. But with tighter control I had more frequent episodes of hypo-glycemia. Three to four times a week the familiar symptoms would wash over me. My heart would start pounding so hard I could feel it in my ears and knees. Everything would go bright until I could no longer distinguish objects, as if a high-intensity light had been turned on in my eyes. Sweat would soak my stomach and the backs of my legs. I'd drink juice, eat candy, anything sweet to pull myself out of the danger zone. The day after an episode of hypoglycemia, my blood sugar rebounded and, in spite of my trying to anticipate it with extra insulin, my heartless monitor would read over three times higher than the normal acceptable range. What had started as a sense of empowerment with my intensive regimen ended in frustration at *my* failure to control dia-betes.

Hypoglycemia is frightening, but when I met Kathy, a twenty-eight-year-old computer-sales coordinator from Pennsylvania, I learned that it pales in comparison to the hor-ror of being diabetic and no longer feeling the early warning symptoms of low blood sugar. Kathy and I had both gone to a seminar on diabetes research held at New York University Hospital. In the outside world, anyone I knew who was diabetic was hiding it as well as I was, but at the seminar, the diabetic people in the audience were openly talking about diabetes and sharing anecdotes. Kathy told me she'd been diabetic since she was seven and had done well on insulin for almost twenty years, but starting in her mid-twenties, she stopped sensing the panicky, sweaty, shaky confusion that warns of low blood sugar. At first the symptoms were delayed, but recently she'd stopped getting symptoms altogether. Every day, quite randomly, all but her vital organs would shut down from sugar deprivation, and she'd black out and fall to the ground. Work was one and a half miles from her home along a road with stoplights and bends and turns; she rarely remembered the drive—not the traffic lights, not the bends in the road, not even other cars. She totaled a car and once ended up in a field. On three other occasions she broke a foot, an ankle, and a knee when her blood sugar dropped too low and she fell.

Over time Kathy lost much of her short-term memory and had to put Post-its on her computer at work to remind herself about team meetings and client presentations. Her body embarrassed her. Every day she was humiliated by the dramatic scenes in which diabetes placed her in the starring role. Instead of the annual salary increases everyone else got, she would get warning letters that she'd lose her job if she were absent anymore. Her performance reviews sounded like medical reports. "I have to do better because without my job I can't afford medical insurance," she had told me with a mix of frustration and despair. "But I don't know what to change because my 'absences' are spent in the emergency room after being scraped off the floor by nine-one-one paramedics."

After trying every combination of insulin, diet, and exercise they could think of, Kathy's doctors advised her not to live alone, to set her alarm clock every few hours through the night to wake her to test her blood sugar, and to give up driving entirely. They wrote "uncontrolled diabetes" in her charts and offered her no hope of getting better. She had looked at me and said, "What am I doing wrong? Everyone else seems to manage. Am I just stupid or something?"

I thought of Kathy when I received a letter from my maternal grandmother—the last one, it turned out, that I'd receive from her. In her youth, Grammy had been a professional ballerina, so she was delighted I had come to New York, the world's arts capital, to go to drama school. Grammy smoked cigarettes that she placed in a long holder and held with her elegant, tapered hands; rarely was she without one. Near the bottom of her letter to me is a small hole with blackened, uneven edges that must have been put there by an ash that fell from the cigarette she was smoking at the time. She had written that she and Grandad were coming to New York, and they wanted to take me to dinner. "We are anxious to see you," she wrote. Then, right under the cigarette burn, she wrote, "Your mother says you haven't been taking very good care of your diabetes. Don't be stupid!"

The letter was postmarked March 16, 1981. Grammy died of angina two days later. By the time I read it she was already gone. What struck me about her letter was that we had never discussed my diabetes. I realized that her last words to me were an echo of the familiar commentary that bounced around behind my back. Essentially she had said that if I couldn't manage diabetes, I was "stupid." And yet Grammy had always supported me in whatever I did, even in my impossible desire for a career in theater and dance. And she was intelligent. If she had known what I knew about diabetes, I am sure she would have rallied to attack the disease rather than me. But how could she have known? I didn't tell her. Diabetics just don't tell.

Chapter 4

The First Complications

Vision, of course, is far more than the collection of light in a photoreceptor. It is also the processing of signals from the visual cells at various stages from the retina to the brain and the final creation of a perception in that poorly understood place we call consciousness.

—*Michael I. Sobel,* Light

From childhood to adolescence and adulthood, diabetes and I were as adversarial and as mutually dependent as a river and the terrain over which it travels. Diabetes molded me while I tried to direct its flow, stopping it from seeping into every crevice of my life by placing boulders in its path. At times I was overwhelmed by its unrelenting permanence, but somewhere along the way, we settled into an uneasy acceptance.

I took insulin with studied regularity. When my blood sugar went up, I took extra; when it went down, I ate. If I couldn't check my blood sugar or was late with a meal, I hoped for the best and ate when I could. I tried to define acceptable parameters for diabetes and to relegate it to a corner where it wouldn't infringe on my ambition and my dreams. I entered that corner only to care for the disease that dwelled there, rarely stopping to ponder my depressed, vulnerable thoughts. From the foregone birthday cakes and thousands of insulin injections to the unscheduled hypoglycemic episodes and craterlike ulcers that appeared on my legs, diabetes intruded in subtle and not so subtle ways. Those closest to me knew that I didn't like to discuss my health and that it infuriated me to be sidelined or singled out by it. I only informed those people who needed to know in the event of a medical emergency. If the subject came up unwittingly I flippantly dismissed it with "insulin, vitamins; everyone takes something. It's no big deal." And of course it wasn't, because I wasn't dealing.

After living with diabetes for fourteen years, I had no signs of secondary complications. Insulin had served me well, taking me from my childhood in England to Virginia, the University of Colorado, theater school in New York, and then back to the University of Colorado, where I graduated with a bachelor's degree in economics. It was then that I returned "home" to Bermuda, to work as a credit analyst at the family bank. Bermuda is an island of plenty, thriving on tourism and exempted insurance business. The coral beaches, guest cottages, and grand old homes in pastel colors sparkle in the white sunlight; colorful birds and flowers punctuate the extravagant greenness. Protected by perilous coral reefs and the great blue Atlantic Ocean, Bermuda has an indigenous immunity to the crime and pollution that plague the world at large.

Mom had come back to Bermuda for a short vacation the

year before and, as with the first time she had visited the island thirty years earlier, married. Her husband, Norman Jones, a long-time friend of our family, had succeeded my paternal grandfather as the chief general manager of the bank. Norman had a modest confidence that steered him calmly through life's calamities. He became both a stabilizing influence in my life and a dear friend.

It felt comfortable to be back in Bermuda, where everything was intrinsically familiar. Each morning I rode my motorbike to the bank along the same road I'd traveled to school as a child. Tony, the little boy who wasn't allowed to eat sweets at my childhood birthday parties, worked at the bank too. Although I saw Tony often, we rarely mentioned diabetes, but I assumed that his desk drawer, like mine, was stocked with insulin, snacks, and a glucose monitor. Every day before lunch, I'd reach into my desk drawer and load my syringe with insulin. When no one was looking I slid the needle through my clothes into my leg or stomach. When small bloody spots occasionally seeped into my shirts and skirts, I just wore my jacket for the rest of the day to cover them up; I don't believe anyone ever noticed.

I was less than six months into my career when I developed an infection in the back of my eye. Concerned it would disrupt my blood sugar control, I went right away to see my childhood eye doctor, Dr. Smith. His hair was silver white now, but he was still in the office I had remembered above the Bermuda Pharmacy with the chart of animals in diminishing sizes hanging on the far wall.

"Do you still have asthma?" he asked.

"Asthma? Gosh, it has been a while hasn't it?"

"The last time I saw you I remember asking if you could

see the purple pig on my eye chart and you said quite seriously, 'No, but I can see the lavender hog.'"

"Well, I'm still a perfectionist but I traded asthma in for diabetes," I explained.

"How long ago was that?" he asked.

"Fourteen years now," I said thinking how much had changed.

He frowned as he looked into my eyes with his beady little light. When he was done, he handed me a prescription for an antibiotic to help fight the infection. I asked him about his daughter, who had been in my class at school before we'd moved to the Bahamas.

"Oh, yes, she is grown now too. I'll tell her you asked about her," he said as he gave me the prescription.

"Thanks a million."

"Deb," he said as I stood to leave, "there's a new eye doctor on the island who's experienced with diabetic eye problems and the most recent advances in caring for them. He has specialized equipment to see the minutest abnormalities. His name is Dr. Hamza, and I'd like you to get an appointment to see him as soon as the infection in your eye is better."

"What's wrong? What did you see?" I asked as I sat back down.

"I only looked in the front of your eyes, but Dr. Hamza will look in the back where any diabetic changes would be noticed. You've had diabetes for fourteen years now, Deb, so it's important to follow you more closely. Most people with diabetes develop what's called nonproliferative or nonhemorrhaging disease of the retina. One third of them never progress beyond that reasonably benign phase, but the rest do get some bleeding in the back of the eye. I don't mean to scare you. Even if there were some changes, they're treatable. I just want you to know what you're up against so you can stay on top of anything that may happen."

"But my vision is terrific," I negotiated. "I could see a bug on the wall of the building across the street!"

"Deb, diabetic retinopathy is often silent. You can't always see it from the inside. You seem in excellent shape to me, so let's hope you're one of the lucky ones. But do your old doctor a favor and go see Dr. Hamza, eh?"

"Okay. Thanks for fitting me in at such short notice, Dr. Smith."

"It's good to see you so well, Deb. You always were the picture of health."

"By the way . . ." I said as I opened the door.

"Yes?"

"I was wrong. The hog is mauve."

Ten days later, I went to see Dr. Hamza. I hated to take the time out in the middle of the workday, but Dr. Smith's cautions had worried me, and I was anxious to get reassurance that I had no diabetic changes. Dr. Hamza dilated my eyes and shone bright lights into what seemed to be the inner sanctum of my brain. The brightness of the lights made tears stream down my face, and my eyes tried to defend themselves by closing in spite of my willing them to cooperate. He held my eyelids open and continued with his examination, pausing several times to draw little X's on his sketch of the anatomy of my eyes. When he was done he turned the lights on, put his instruments down, and calmly told me that I had microaneurysms in the blood vessels in my eyes, indicating the very early stages of diabetic retinopathy.

I tried to talk him out of his diagnosis. "Are you sure?

How can that be? I've never had any eye trouble. My vision is perfect! Nothing's changed about my diabetes. Why would they start now?"

"Deb, the diabetic changes in the tiny blood vessels throughout the body, microvascular changes, start very early in diabetes, but the symptoms can take years to show up. These changes occur in the eyes of eighty percent of the diabetic population after only fifteen years of living with the disease. For you the chances were higher because twenty-six percent of those who have insulin-dependent diabetes have these changes within the first ten years. You're doing very well, Deb. The changes are small and we've caught them early."

So what if I was doing slightly better than average, I thought. Fourteen, twenty, ten years, what difference did it make? I had developed complications. As quickly as the ominous thought entered my head, I tried to conquer it with optimism and disbelief. "My great-grandmother and great-uncle were diabetic, and they never had any eye trouble. Nor does Uncle Dick, and he's diabetic too. Complications don't run in my family!"

"Deb, don't be overly concerned. As long as you continue to keep your blood sugars under control and get regular checkups, everything should be okay. For the time being, I'm going to refer you for a new treatment that is very effective at slowing the progression of retinopathy."

"From progressing to what?" I asked, as if the horrifying statistics I'd read about the relationship between diabetes and blindness were only fund-raising propaganda. The truth was, Dr. Hamza was talking about *me*, and no amount of academic understanding could bridge that gulf between impersonal facts and personal experience.

"Diabetes weakens the retinal blood vessels and restricts circulation, causing a reduced supply of oxygen to the retina, the screen of nerves at the back of the eye that helps to send images to the brain. New blood vessels form to carry oxygen to the oxygen-deprived parts. At first they appear as small protrusions in the vessel walls; these are the microaneurysms I see in the back of your eyes. If they're left untreated, they can proliferate and form a fragile web of new vessels that are susceptible to rupturing, causing the hemorrhaging that can lead to severe vision loss. By treating your eyes before this process gets under way, we can probably prevent this from getting too much worse."

"How do you treat them?" I asked urgently.

"Well, we can't do it here yet because we don't have the equipment. You'll have to go to Boston, where they recently started using laser technology to treat diabetic eye diseases. What they do is shoot a narrow, high-energy beam of light through the pupil to create numerous small, relatively harmless scars on the retina. Killing small patches of the retina reduces the requirement for oxygen and substantially limits the risk of hemorrhaging in the new blood vessels. You can do this as an outpatient. The treatment itself is uncomfortable but not painful."

"I don't care how uncomfortable it is, I just want it fixed!" I said bluntly.

"You're going to be fine, Deb. We've really caught this very early on. The key is, from now on, to have someone look into the back of your eyes three times a year and, most importantly, for you to keep your blood sugar under control."

"Will you give me a guarantee?"

He evaded me with a smile. "Nothing in life is guaranteed.

I'd like you to make an appointment as soon as possible with Dr. Lloyd Aiello at the Joslin Diabetes Center in Boston. Dr. Aiello is one of the pioneers of this new treatment. Plan to stay for several days," he said putting his hand on my shoulder. "Oh, and be very careful not to lift anything heavy, and don't lean over. You want to avoid pressure in your eyes. You'll need to sleep at a forty-five degree angle too, okay?"

"I'll do whatever it takes," I sighed.

I wanted to believe Dr. Hamza when he said my eyes would be all right, yet the realization that I had developed a secondary complication of diabetes frightened me. Repeatedly I'd wake up from a nightmare in which I was a child again, blindfolded and swinging at the snowman piñata. Then someone would take the blindfold off and I still couldn't see. I was stuck in a room and couldn't find the door. When I woke up I'd turn on the light by my bed and just lie there imagining what it would be like to be blind. I requested a week of vacation time, knowing that taking time off after only five months at my new job was sending management a misleading message about my work ethic, but I worried that the truth would cause them greater concern about my long-term productivity. I chose to table my anxiety about work and fly to Boston for my "vacation" to get those "numerous, relatively harmless, small scars on my retinas to protect my vision." Mom insisted on accompanying me.

The winter of 1984 was the worst the Northeast had seen in decades. After our flight descended into Boston's snow-covered Logan International Airport and pulled up to the gate, Mom and the other passengers around me jumped up and inched toward the door at the front of the aircraft. I waited; I was in no rush to embrace my premonition that at twenty-four my healthy years were waning. As the stragglers headed for the exit I took my small carry-on bag from the overhead compartment and followed Mom off the plane. My sister Lesley, by then a physical therapist living in Boston and working in the orthopedic department at Massachusetts General Hospital, was there to meet us. As we drove west on Storrow Drive, I watched enviously as joggers puffed along the icy banks of the Charles. High above the road, the red brick townhouses sat like spectators at a parade. The salt covered road turned up and to the left and from there I could see the small collection of skyscrapers in Boston's financial district. We turned onto Boylston Street and then through an intersection to Longwood Avenue.

Longwood Avenue was the Wall Street of hospitals: there was Brigham and Women's, Beth Israel, Children's, New England Deaconess, and the Joslin Diabetes Center. Joslin is one of the world's pre-eminent and oldest clinics specializing in diabetes. Dr. Elliott Joslin had begun treating diabetic patients there in 1898. Because he was one of the two leading diabetologists at the beginning of the 1900s, his was one of the first clinics to get supplies of insulin after its introduction in Toronto in 1922. Doctors in their white and green attire hurried between buildings along with other staff members: nurses, cleaning people, technicians, physical therapists, social workers, administrators, pharmacists, rabbis, priests, charity workers, and students—all of them with intense purpose in their carriage as they managed their pieces of the complex machine of medicine.

Dr. Hamza had been right that the laser treatments didn't hurt, but the anticipation of holding my face pressed up against the machine, knowing that the laser beams shooting through my pupils would burn and scar my retina, made me break out in a cold sweat. The treatments lasted only ten to fifteen minutes each, but five hundred burns were made each time. My eyes needed to be treated one quadrant at a time with three days to heal between sessions, so my few days in Boston became a few weeks. My eyes were dilated and sensitive to light after each treatment. The glare on the snow combined with the neuropathy in my feet made me totally dependent on Mom to lead me through the snow to the bus stop where we'd catch a bus back to Lesley's home in Marblehead. Each time the healing period was over we'd return to Longwood Avenue for another round of treatment. We'd sit in the waiting room at the eye clinic, surrounded by diabetic people in wheelchairs with patches on their eyes and orthopedic shoes on their feet. As I waited for my turn behind the menacing steel machine I felt disengaged from those people with their complications. My treatments, I told myself, were preventive: I was fortunate I wasn't a severe diabetic like they were.

When I returned to Joslin for my follow-up appointment six months later, my doctors were amazed by how well my eyes had responded to the laser burns. The microaneurysms had disappeared completely. Apart from limiting my depth perception, no permanent damage had been done. More resolute than ever that I would beat the odds, I returned to my normal, everyday diabetic routine and dismissed retinopathy as a minor, isolated episode. Little did I know that I was heeding Ovid's instruction: "Live," says Death, "for I am coming."

Chapter 5

Small Patches of Numbness

I ask not for valor,
Since deformity is daring.
It is its essence to o'ertake mankind
By heart and soul, and make itself the equal—
Ay, the superior of the rest. There is
A spur in its halt movements, to become
All that the others cannot, in such things
As still are free to both, to compensate
For stepdame Nature's avarice at first.
—*Lord Byron, "The Deformed Transformed"*

After I worked for several years as a credit analyst at the small bank in Bermuda, the fast-paced, ambitious energy of New York City beckoned. I moved away from the peaceful, relaxed little island in the Atlantic to be a researcher at the executive search firm on Park Avenue. When the firm went out of business a few years later, I went out on my own as an independent consultant, traveling for two weeks of every month. My father, always standing by with his quiet support, helped me to buy a small apartment on New York's Upper East Side. Having my own apartment made me feel grounded, like I belonged somewhere. Although it had a breathtaking view of the city for thirty blocks to the south, the apartment was generically bland and boxy. I launched into a project to convert it into a clean and colorful refuge from the bustle and filth of the city. On weekends I devoted many afternoon hours to what became my second obsession, the meticulous renovation of my home. I sponge-painted the walls with rich, natural colors, made curtains, added cornice moldings, and replaced closet doors and doorknobs. There is no better distraction from one obsession than indulging in another, and so it was that my life migrated back and forth between work and painting, work and hammering, work and sanding, and going to hardware stores.

I had all but forgotten my minor bout with retinopathy. Diabetes was no more than an annoyance to fit in around my active and healthy life. When the first signs of neuropathy started, I thought that the discomfort in my legs was merely a strained muscle or some other normal occurrence. But when the discomfort intensified and became shooting pains that felt as though my nerves had been plugged into an electrical outlet, I grew suspicious that I was again under attack by diabetes. At night helpless tears dampened my pillow as the pain played up and down my legs. No aspirin or codeine could stop the agony. I'd lie staring at the ceiling, begging for sleep. You don't feel pain when you're sleeping.

Over time the pain went away and was replaced by small patches of numbness on the outside of my knees and shins. These patches spread and connected, and by the fall my legs were numb below my knees. They could no longer warn me of hot or cold, of broken toes or of blisters. I pleaded for my pain to return—but the numbness marched on. Refusing to believe that neuropathy was a symptom of a progressive and insidious decline that had been underway for years, I blamed myself for not exercising enough and for not controlling my blood sugar well enough. I started exercising compulsively, checking my blood sugar eight or more times a day, and eating precise measurements of plain foods whose exact number of grams of protein, carbohydrate, and fat I could calculate. I kept tapping my knees and putting my feet in hot and cold water to see if the neuropathy was improving. Somehow I always managed to conclude that it was. Yet the nerves in my legs were dying, and my feet were getting weaker. By the middle of the summer of 1989, the nerves in my ankles that should have given me a sense, or awareness, of my body's position had been all but lost to diabetes' attack. Messages from the proprioceptors in my feet no longer reached my brain to tell me I was falling. It seemed that the more I concentrated on walking straight, the more I'd stagger into walls and furniture. Often I'd trip when my toes didn't clear the ground. For several months my knees had open, infected wounds from being grazed repeatedly.

I went to the library to search for new information, or a sign of hope, but everything I read said there were no effective treatments for neuropathy. Worse, I learned that diabetic neuropathy often attacks the automatic functions of the body, masking the warning signs of dangerously low blood-sugar levels, and causing erratic digestion. I kept reading, hoping to find answers, but instead I found worse truths about diabetes. The reality left me in despair, terrified at the prospect of helplessly watching as my disease slowly and surely violated my body. Then came the moment when I had walked out of my shoe, and found myself a block from home wearing only one. I had decided then to get a cane, "just for a while, until my feet improved." And so, my trip to Brooks Brothers.

"I'm looking for a cane," I said to the aloof and patronizing salesperson.

"Whom is it for?" he asked as he beckoned me to follow him.

"Well, it's for me," I admitted, adding quickly, "I'm recuperating from a skiing accident."

"Ours are rather expensive for temporary use," he sniffed, "but I'll show you what we have."

There were five to choose from—not five kinds—five. So I picked one in natural rosewood with a comfortable and unusual handgrip.

"I'll take this one. How much is it?" I asked.

"It's three hundred dollars."

"Oh. They are expensive, aren't they?" I hesitated. "Well, I guess it's an investment in the future. They'll probably cost ten times as much by the time I'm ninety and then I'll be glad I already have one." He indulged me with a dry, faint smile.

"It's too long for you," he said flatly.

"How can you tell?"

"Your arm is overly bent when you hold it, as if you were holding a staff, not a cane. You won't get any leverage from it when you go up stairs."

"Oh," I paused. "Can I get it cut shorter?"

"Of course, but then you'll need to change the tip. You should get a rubber tip so it doesn't slip when it's raining and the sidewalks are wet."

"Where would I get tips for a cane?"

"At the drugstore," he said as if he were talking to a halfwit. He wrapped the cane in brown paper and I stumbled home without using it.

A few days later, one of my father's clients, an investment company in Bermuda, called to ask me to recruit a Bermudian partner from North America. The discussion led to a retained assignment. When I flew "home" to go over the

details, I left my cane in New York. I wasn't doing as well
with diabetes as my uncle was, and I didn't want word to get
around the small, entwined community that I was having
trouble. Each day that I was there lunch was delayed, and
when I went to the ladies room to hide in a stall to check my
blood, my glucose level was always too low. To avoid having
insulin reactions, while I waited for everyone else to be ready
for lunch I'd sip cups of coffee with three sugars. By then my
sugar level would be too high to eat, so I'd settle for a salad
and just eat the lettuce.

The island's small local newspaper heard that I had
started a consulting business to help repatriate Bermudians
to local businesses, so they called me for an interview.
Their article used "my story" with all its spin about how I
preferred the entrepreneur's life of working with low overhead, by and for myself from "an office in my home." Even
my friends and relatives bought into the charade, telling
each other about what an inspiration I was, what a positive
attitude I had, and about how I had conquered diabetes.
They didn't see the diabetic's smokescreen that I had engineered to rationalize a career choice motivated by necessity.

One day toward the end of the summer, I decided to cheer
up my gloomy, windowless kitchen by power-sanding and
freshening up the heavy, paint-encrusted cabinets there. The
project sorely tested my ability to balance because I needed
to use both my hands to stop the power sander from spinning
out of control. I found that by using my elbows and knees for
stability, I could compensate for my senseless nerves. I developed confidence by mastering control of the sander on the
lower cabinets, then clambered onto the counter to complete
the job on the ones hung high above. Touching the wall with

my elbows or knees, I threw myself into clearing one circular patch of about a foot in diameter after another.

After completing the outsides of the cabinets, and delighted with my work, I climbed down to rest my arms and to have a glass of water. Suddenly, I was aware of the strange and acrid smell of cooking meat mingled with old paint and wood. I couldn't imagine where the meat smell came from because I hadn't cooked in my kitchen for weeks. I went over to my sofa to lie down for a minute, but when I looked down at my feet my stomach turned at the sight of blood and fluid soaking through the sock on my left foot. The smell grew stronger, and the bile rose in the back of my throat as I realized what had happened. I'd been standing on the counter in the kitchen with one foot touching the stove, and my toe must have been over the pilot light. I hadn't realized that my neuropathy was that bad, preventing me from heeding the white-hot warning that should have made me pull away in time. How could I not have felt my own flesh being burned?

At that moment the "hows" and "whys" didn't matter. I knew that I had to get to a doctor to try to fight back the bacteria that would already be reveling in the tissues of my glucose-enriched body. Infection and diabetes form a vicious cycle. Bacteria thrive in glucose, and infection elevates blood sugar levels, making diabetes control elusive. If this infection were to go beyond the control of antibiotics, I could lose my toe, or even my foot. I knew the dangers only too well. I'd been hospitalized before with diabetic ulcers, areas where the skin disintegrates and opens like craters that expand and can turn gangrenous. Many of the patients on the vascular floors where I'd been admitted were diabetics recovering from amputations caused when this process outran the most potent antibiotics. Without taking the time to test my blood sugar, I put a slipper on my injured foot and called my vascular specialist. I had so many doctors that I'd put them all in the "D" section of my address book in case I forgot their names. Among others, I had a primary care physician, an ophthalmologist, an optometrist, a kidney specialist, a vascular specialist, a podiatrist, an infectious disease specialist, and a dietitian.

As I suspected he would, the doctor cleaned out the hole in my toe, packed it with gauze dipped in antibacterial liquid, and prescribed large doses of antibiotics. After wrapping my foot in bandages, carefully avoiding getting tape on my parchmentlike skin, he sent me home with a big, wooden-soled orthopedic shoe and instructions to stay off my foot except to go to the bathroom. I was to cleanse and pack the wound several times a day and to return to his office in five days unless I noticed redness, oozing, or swelling before then. I silently reviewed every possible subterfuge so I could continue with my consulting assignments while, at the same time, avoid walking so my toe could heal. This was one of the times I recognized the value of my home office because I could manage without anyone knowing what had happened.

Throughout the nights and days that followed, I practiced the "sick day" rules of diabetes; pricking my finger every three or four hours, day and night, to squeeze out the little drop of blood that would help me decide whether or not to eat and how much, if any, additional insulin I should inject. To the outside world my work appeared to be going on as usual. The Black Monday stock market disaster twenty months earlier had sparked massive lay-offs on Wall Street and had undermined the confidence of graduate students who called, nervously presenting their credentials. While I interviewed and negotiated with them, and settled training

issues with the companies that would teach them to be brokers, diabetes, the Hyde in my Jekyll-and-Hyde life of disease
and health, tormented me behind the scenes. With derisive
amusement, I smiled at the image of myself in shorts and T-
shirt, a sock on one foot and bandages on the other, squeez-
ing blood from my finger for testing while I talked to people
all over the world about their careers in brokerage. I'd
respond to their sociable "How are you?" greetings with a
perfunctory "great" and quickly segue to a topic of interest to
the caller.

On the morning of my follow-up doctor's appointment I
noticed redness and swelling when I went to change the ban-
dage. I knew right away that I was in for a long battle and my
spirits plummeted. How could a hole in one small toe cause
so much trouble? With a feeling of foreboding, I went to the
doctor who, as soon as he saw my toe, told me I would need
to be admitted to the hospital. Because the Joslin Diabetes
Center in Boston knew my history, I called there and was
admitted to the vascular floor of the adjoining New England
Deaconess Hospital. My admission papers read:

> "Type 1 IDDM (insulin-dependent diabetes mellitus)
> Retinopathy
> Neuropathy
> Hypertension [the first signs of kidney disease]
> . . . pronounced peripheral neuropathy with impaired sen-
> sation to ankles and absent position sense in her feet. Her
> gait was wide based. On plantar surface of her left first toe
> she had a well-healed ulcer. Initial X-rays of her left foot
> showed irregularity of the cortex on the medial aspect of
> her left third toe not excluding osteomyelitis [bone infec-
> tion]."

After several consultations and more X-rays, it was unanimous; the infection had indeed spread to my bone, and a section of my toe would have to be removed to avoid losing my foot. The surgeon used only a mild anesthetic, yet physically I didn't feel a thing. What I did feel was rage and frustration: frustration because such a simple human act as wearing socks to stand on the counter in my kitchen had elicited lectures about how diabetics must always wear shoes, as if I, not diabetes, were the guilty party. And I was angry, angry because half of my toe had to be cut off because diabetes had killed it. Diabetes had taken a quantifiable piece of me away.

While I recuperated I continued to work from the hospital without letting anyone know I was there. To send faxes I wheeled myself down to the Mail Boxes Etc. store near the entrance to Joslin. When I couldn't reach someone by phone I'd leave a message saying, "I'm on the road at the moment, I'll call back in a while." The public address system in the hospital sounded just like that of an airport and I don't believe any of my clients noticed the difference. It was several days after the surgery that the managing director of the Asian subsidiaries of my brokerage client called to invite me to make a presentation at the annual management meeting in London. The meeting was to be the following week. It couldn't be worse timing, I thought as I glared at my bandaged foot, which was propped up on a pillow at the end of the bed. Estimating that I could be up and about in a few days, I accepted the engagement in London. From the phone in my hospital room, I booked a flight and a hotel, and began negotiating my discharge. It grated on me to have to wait for doctor's orders to continue with my life, like a child asking for permission to go out and play. The doctor would never have agreed to my plan if he'd known that it included going to London. So, having long since learned that debating with the medical profession about the relative importance of events in my life only served to frustrate all of us, I kept my travel plans to myself. Because ultimately the decisions were mine, I charted my course with diabetes as a part of my life, rather than as my entire life. The attending physician ordered the discontinuation of the IV antibiotics and discharged me on oral antibiotics three days before I was scheduled to go overseas.

An electric cart drove me to the departure gate at the airport, and another picked me up when we landed. I was wearing a clunky orthopedic shoe on my left foot and a sneaker on my right, though I'd packed a pair of professional shoes to wear for my presentation. It was only 8:00 in the morning when I limped out into the cool, moist air at Heathrow airport, just outside London. Because of my childhood in England I felt a sense of safety there. A cheerful cabby jumped out of his boxy, high-riding black taxi and opened one of the reverse-engineered doors for me. As the distinctive diesel engine chugged along the motorway into London, he chatted merrily through the dividing window.

"What 'appened to yer foot there, luv?"

"Ah, I broke my toe."

"How'd you do that then?"

"Um, I, uh, my horse stood on it." *Oh, please!* I thought to myself. I would have to do better than that if I was to get through the next few days.

Just before my meeting, I slipped my feet into a pair of low-heeled, black leather pumps, loving the way my ankles looked so pretty and flawless and picturing my feet as they had been before this grotesque chapter with diabetes had begun. As I walked to the podium to make my presentation, nobody knew about my broken and burned toes or the scarring in the back of my eyes from retinopathy and laser surgery. Nor did they know that I pushed needles into my body nine or more times a day to administer insulin and draw blood. They didn't see my hands trembling as my blood sugar started to drop. And *I* didn't remember what I said, or indeed how I got back to my hotel room.

The next morning I went to meet with the managing director. Still unsure of what he had meant the day before on the phone about my "spectacular performance," I asked forthrightly, "How did I do?"

"As I said, you were spectacular. In fact, after you left, I got five requests for assignments for you from our offices in Asia. That's why I wanted to meet with you this morning. We need to go over the job specifications, so you can get started." For the next hour I listened intently and made notes about the assignments. As we stood to leave he said, "Deb, are you feeling better today? You seemed a little tired yesterday."

"Never felt better. Yesterday the jet lag got to me."

Chapter 6

Circling the Drain

You can be an expert surfer and hit the perfect ninth wave, but if the tide is going out, that wave, no matter how big, will not reach the beach.

—Julian Snyder, introduction to
The Long Wave Cycle *by Nikolai Kondratieff*

Seventy-five years ago Elizabeth Hughes, the daughter of the secretary of state under Warren G. Harding, was dying of diabetes. When her mother, Antoinette, read about insulin, the experimental and promising new treatment that had been developed in Toronto, she wrote directly to Dr. Banting to ask about insulin for her daughter. His reply said simply that insulin was still in its experimental stages—an unacceptable answer for a mother trying to save her daughter's life. With dogged determination, Antoinette Hughes appealed the decision and, before long, word came back that Elizabeth would be one of the first people to be treated with insulin. The question then wasn't "What will happen if Elizabeth tries insulin?" but "What will happen if she doesn't?" By the age of fourteen, only two years after her diagnosis with diabetes, Elizabeth had wasted away to a mere forty-five pounds. Intuitively, without analyzing the risks, Elizabeth grabbed the lifeline and was rewarded with fifty-five additional years of life.

Sixty years later, at the end of the 1980s, I had lived a full and happy twenty years using insulin. I had my bouts with both diabetic eye and nerve disease, but had never stopped to think that those complications were part of a steady progression. But Mom was watching me run harder and harder to stay in the same place. She knew that the rosy picture of diabetes that we had been shown over the years was turning into a crimson warning. One day she read an article about pancreas transplantation, an experimental and promising new procedure that had actually freed some people who had been insulin-dependent diabetics since childhood! The article said that of the more than 2,500 pancreas transplants that had been performed worldwide, more than half had been done here in the United States. Just as Antoinette Hughes had done when she first heard about insulin, Mom called her endocrinologist, desperate to find a cure for me. She told the doctor that I'd been diabetic for twenty years and that every year there were more diabetic complications, with no sign that things would get better.

"She's only in her twenties!" Mom explained and then, hopefully, she asked, "I read an article about pancreas transplants and wonder if this might be an answer for my daughter?"

"Does she have kidney disease?" the doctor asked.

"No, thank heavens," Mom sighed.

The physician paused and then went on to explain that pancreas transplants were experimental, reserved only for people who already needed kidney transplants.

"If Deborah ever needs to think about having a kidney transplant it would make sense to look into the possibility of getting a pancreas too. The reason it's done this way is that immunosuppression drugs, the lifelong regimen of medicines required to prevent the rejection of transplanted organs, have side effects. If your daughter needed a kidney, she would need to take these drugs anyway to protect the new kidney. It would make perfect sense then to be free of diabetes too. Sara, the question is really, "Which is worse, diabetes or transplant surgery and immunosuppression?"

"What are the side effects of the drugs?" Mom asked.

The doctor told her about the risk of serious infections and the 1 percent increased risk of lymphoma. There could be cosmetic changes too, she explained, such as excess hair growth or puffy cheeks. She explained that transplant recipients needed to take steroids and how, over time, steroids often caused bone weakness, leading to hip replacements. And then, of course, a transplant would be major surgery. There were always risks with surgery.

"But now she's at risk for severe vision loss, amputation, and kidney disease; she's already on that path. Why wait for her health to get worse? Why put her through more? What if she goes blind or something irreversible happens? Why not try to prevent kidney disease?" Mom rationalized. "My daughter's not going to get better on insulin—nobody's said there's a chance of that. I've got to do something. . . ."

"I wish I had an answer for you, Sara," the doctor said sympathetically. "Every year immunosuppression drugs improve.

Maybe there will be something better soon. Try to wait a little longer."

Mom had watched as laser beams were shot into my eyes thousands of times to slow the progression of diabetic retinopathy, and again several years later when streaks of blood tracked across my vision. She witnessed my desperate anger as my ability to walk was distorted by neuropathy, and she had seen my gradual loss of dignity and withdrawal from society—but my kidneys continued to function normally. Mom, the woman who believed that every story should have a happy ending, kept asking "Why wait?" only to be told, "Deborah isn't sick enough yet." And so she continued to watch my health deteriorate—half hoping that my kidneys would fail so I could get a kidney and pancreas transplant.

All I knew about transplants was what I'd seen in the media: "Liver Transplant: Desperate Attempt to Save Life" and "Child Will Die If New Heart Not Found." When Mom told me about her conversation with her doctor I thought, *You've got to be kidding! I'm not dying! I'd much rather take insulin than have a transplant!* I believed that with insulin I could stay healthy long enough to benefit when a cure was found. And so I continued to wait for *the* cure that had been "right around the corner" since the early 1900s—all the while believing that the worst of the complications were over. All I have to do, I thought, is to control my blood sugar. So I'd keep setting new rules: exercise before dinner instead of before breakfast; pack the same lunch every day; set my alarm to check my blood sugar at 3:00 A.M.; eat more fiber; take more vitamin B. . . . There was always something that I needed to do to control my diabetes.

I didn't view my experiences with retinopathy and neuropathy on a continuum, as part of a progressive disease process. I had had retinopathy, and laser surgery had fixed it—period. But of course retinopathy can't be cured with laser surgery because the damage is caused by diabetes, and laser surgery can't cure diabetes. I remained staunchly optimistic that with good blood-sugar control and regular visits to the ophthalmologist, retinopathy would no longer be a problem. Each time Band-Aids were put on the symptoms of diabetes I'd say to myself, "If this is the worst that ever happens to me, I'll be fine." It was part of the same psychological disconnect that had me believing I was different from *those* diabetics in the waiting room at Joslin with their orthopedic shoes, eye patches, and wheelchairs.

Not long after that *I* had an orthopedic shoe, and *I* had needed a cane to walk. As the months passed, my neuropathy worsened and the downward trend of my health became patently obvious. There was no more denying that I was deteriorating; not gradually, but one system right after another. The neuropathy that had started out in the peripheral nerves of my legs spread to the nerves that controlled my automatic functions. This "autonomic neuropathy" caused "gastroparesis," an inability to digest properly. Undigested food and acid collected in my stomach and frequently made me vomit with no warning. I tried to adjust my insulin doses to compensate for my erratic digestion but there was no way to know how much, or when, the carbohydrates and proteins I ate would be converted to glucose. It was a gruesome roller coaster ride between the troughs of hypoglycemia and the peaks of hyperglycemia.

In the summer of 1990, too sick from diabetes to be at home yet too well to be in the hospital, I was again admitted to the Joslin Diabetes Center. Joslin was a cross between a college dormitory and a hospital, and over the years it had become a refuge for me. Gastroparesis had completely undermined my attempts to control my blood-sugar levels; I knew that the doctors at Joslin could help me. Everything was institutionalized and, for a while, I felt as if my diabetes could be controlled. It was the doctors at Joslin who had saved my vision, and it was here that I had lost my toe to save my foot. Meals were punctual, the food simple, the portions precise. Nurses drifted in and out during the night to check my blood-sugar levels; four-ounce cups of apple juice would materialize at 3:00 A.M. to prevent my blood sugar from going too low during the night. At Joslin I felt safe.

Every day doctors lectured in the auditorium on managing and living with diabetes. They spoke about peak and trough reaction times of various types of insulin; diabetic complications; understanding FDA labeling on food packages; calculating carbohydrate and protein grams; dining out; calculating insulin doses when traveling across time zones; treating hypo- and hyperglycemic episodes; managing sick days; and on and on. Always I looked forward to the research lecture, hoping to hear some validation of my tenuous hopes that a cure would be found in my lifetime; but the talk of wonderful advances in nasal insulin research, noninvasive blood-glucose monitors and needleless insulin guns fell flat on my ears. The problem is *diabetes*, I thought. Why are we learning more and more about managing the symptoms instead of concentrating on curing the underlying disease?

The doctors at Joslin were concerned about the apparent worsening of my condition. Right away they ordered blood and urine tests to see how well my kidneys were filtering toxins from my body. At birth, healthy kidneys are capable of filtering 120 milliliters of creatinine per minute; with each passing year their filtration rate is reduced by one milliliter per minute. Creatinine, the end product of the metabolism of an amino acid found in muscles and blood, is used as the indicator of kidney function. First the concentration of creatinine was measured in my blood and then the rate at which it was filtered by my kidneys was determined by the amount of creatinine evident in a twenty-four-hour urine collection. By comparing that information with the results of prior tests, the doctor could estimate how fast my kidneys were deteriorating and how much longer they could be expected to function.

Beginning with my first instance of diabetic complications in 1984, every visit to the doctor had, without exception, left me with more restrictions and less optimism about my future health. There had been a tectonic shift from the old banalities of "You'll live a normal and healthy life" to "Complications after this many years of diabetes can only be expected." And so it was during my consultation with the nephrologist about the results of my kidney function tests. After his cursory greeting he said quite casually, "It looks to me like your kidneys should function for another four years at this rate."

I was twenty-nine.

Didn't he know what kidney failure would mean to me? I wondered if he, who saw so many diabetic people with kidney disease, thought I was just one more noncompliant diabetic who had brought this on herself. Indeed, I wondered if in fact I had.

"Diabetic kidney disease, or nephropathy, is very common after twenty years on insulin, and it certainly explains all the symptoms you're having—edema in your ankles, low red blood count, fatigue, and elevated blood pressure." He seemed not the least bit surprised that I had eye disease, nerve disease, and now this.

So there it was. Diabetic kidney disease is progressive. The die had been cast. I would end up on dialysis and with a kidney transplant; it was just a matter of time. As my thoughts wandered through dark passages, the doctor droned on about prescriptions for blood-pressure medication and a consultation with a dietitian about a new "renal" diet.

A few years earlier when I had been admitted to the vascular floor across the street at the New England Deaconess Hospital, I had been roaming the halls in my wheelchair to get some exercise, and I saw "Dialysis Unit" on one of the doors. I was drawn in by a need to confront my fear of kidney failure, to embrace the downside, and to know that if it happened I could cope; but I had only confirmed my fear. The dialysis unit was one of the saddest places I'd ever seen. I could picture it vividly now. People lying on narrow cots covered in blankets as tubes sucked the blood from their bodies and ran it through machines to purify it before returning it to them. The room smelled of a pungent blend of sick people, disinfectant, and dialysis fluid. Most of the people in there had diabetes—their faces resigned and void of emotion as if they had surrendered to their disease. As I witnessed those slaves to science, it seemed to me that there was little difference between dialysis and death.

"There are a number of things you can do to slow the progression," my doctor said as he handed me several prescriptions. "Most importantly you need to keep your blood pressure under control. Those prescriptions you're holding are for two types of diuretics and a blood-pressure medication. You're carrying a good ten pounds of excess fluid. Getting rid of it will help your blood pressure. Also, I want you to check your blood pressure several times a day; perhaps the easiest way would be to do it when you check your blood sugar and take insulin."

"And what about my day job?" I said, from behind my screen of bravado.

"We're always looking for good nurses," he said with a hint of a smile. "I'll send the dietitian in to tell you about the 'renal' diet. Then I'll be back and we can talk."

The dietitian told me to avoid potassium and phosphorous whenever possible, to stay away from drinks with caffeine and to stop eating tomatoes, bananas, oranges, potatoes, and cheese. My daily allowance of protein was cut to thirty-five grams per day. That meant no protein at breakfast and two ounces of meat at lunch and dinner. Two ounces of chicken is about three large bites, simply not enough to satisfy my hunger. The "renal" diet reduced my intake in all the food groups except fat, so I was to use butter and cream cheese to keep my calorie count up. I felt as though I was blindfolded, trying to control a car with only the brakes and accelerator while the steering wheel had been commandeered by diabetes.

Searching for consolation, I asked the doctor when he returned, "If I need a new kidney could I get a new pancreas and be cured of diabetes too?"

"Maybe in the next few years we'll talk about getting you a new kidney, but don't worry about that now."

"And what about a pancreas? I can get a pancreas too, right?"

"No, Deb. Pancreas transplants are experimental and there are all sorts of problems with them. We know that intensive management with insulin can really reduce the risk of your complications progressing, so let's stick with that."

"But the problem is that it isn't the intensive *management* that helps with complications, it's getting good blood-sugar levels that matters. I can't tell you how frustrated I am that I can't translate intensive management into good results."

"I know it's difficult, Deb, but I'd strongly advise you to continue as you are until something better than pancreas transplants comes along."

My doctors had never steered me wrong. They had always been there to fix the ulcers on my legs, protect my vision, help me through the flu. They had even sustained me through a ruptured appendix. "It's just so hard to learn that my efforts over the years were insufficient," I reflected.

"You're doing well for someone who's had diabetes as long as you have. Look at all the things you are able to do in your work and travel. You'll be all right. You remind me of a patient who I told eight years ago that her kidneys would fail in three years."

"Why do I remind you of her?" I asked hopefully.

"Because like you, she works on Wall Street and travels all over the world for her job. By managing her blood sugar and blood pressure and following the 'renal' diet, she was able to delay dialysis until just six months ago. She doesn't let anything stop her. She takes her dialysis equipment to work with her and gets it sent in advance to the hotels she's staying in. She's waiting for a new kidney, and I'm sure she won't miss a beat with that either."

"How do people manage?" I asked rhetorically as I pictured the young woman sitting in an office in downtown New York with bags of dialysis fluid dripping through a surgically implanted tube in her abdomen. I didn't want to be like her. I wanted to be free of disease and needles and tubes—and doctors. I thought back to all the times when as a child I'd heard the likes of "Science is moving so fast, 'they' will find answers in time," or "They couldn't put men on the moon when you were born. Stay healthy so you can benefit from the cure when it is found." Here I was, just one month shy of my twentieth anniversary with diabetes and, just as the statistics had warned I might, I had joined the 30 percent of diabetics who succumb to kidney failure after twenty years with the disease.

When I called Mom and told her about my prognosis, the little seed of hope she had protected all those years burst open. "Sweetie, maybe some good will come of all this. If you have kidney disease, you can get a new pancreas and be cured of diabetes at the same time, you know. I have the name and some phone numbers for one of the leading pancreas-transplant surgeons in the world, Dr. Hans Sollinger; he's in Wisconsin. Why don't you call him?" she asked, knowing that I hated to discuss diabetes, but struggling to find answers for a disease that she felt was hers too.

I explained what my doctor had thought about pancreas transplants and with resignation said, "Mom, there have been too many doctors. I need to get back to my life. This diabetes is consuming me psychologically and physically. Don't worry, I can overcome this. I'm just feeling a little low right now."

"Take the phone numbers and call him when you want to. I've talked to him. He is one of the best transplant surgeons in the world. You'll get along well with him. He wants to help."

"Thanks, Mom." I wrote the numbers on a small piece of paper and after hanging up the phone I put it on my dresser. But I couldn't bring myself to call. Every time I looked at that piece of paper I'd remember my nephrologist in Boston and how adamant he had been about the dangers. What if they each saw my options differently? Whose advice would I take? The doctor at Joslin or the one in Wisconsin? Both of them were leading experts on diabetes. *Maybe this is all a pipe dream,* I thought. If a pancreas transplant could get rid of diabetes, then why weren't diabetics around the world clamoring for this new remedy? The very idea that a doctor in Wisconsin had cured several hundred diabetics without making headline news was as absurd as thinking that cancer or AIDS could be cured without the media knowing about it!

Every day I looked at the piece of paper on my dresser wondering what would help me make my decision. I replayed the words of the doctor at Joslin over and over. "Your kidney disease is early on yet. . . . another four years . . . you remind me of her . . . she was able to delay dialysis until six months ago . . . check your blood pressure, take diuretics and blood pressure medication, follow a 'renal' diet, take insulin, test your blood sugar and then maybe you can delay . . . nephropathy isn't reversible. . . ." My health was crumbling ever faster as I battled through days of throwing up in taxis and stumbling on the streets with my cane. Before long I slipped to yet another new low and had to be fitted with braces so I could walk.

The moment that helped me decide was when one of my clients called and asked me to do an assignment in Europe.

For the first time ever I declined, because I knew that physically I couldn't do the work. I didn't decline because I had had a temporary setback. I declined because, even on a good day, I couldn't do the work. The path I was on could, at best, delay dialysis—but that was all. With my horizons imploding, I went to call the number on the little piece of paper that had sat on my dresser for over a year.

The frustration and unfulfilled hope of twenty-two years stuck in my throat as Dr. Sollinger explained the benefits and the risks of surgery, as well as the secondary complications of the drugs required to prevent the rejection of transplanted organs. Nevertheless, I liked his confidence and his way of putting the process in the context of my hopes and dreams. Tears started rolling down my face and dropping in little pools on the pad I had planned to write notes on. There were no notes to write because I had no questions. Perhaps in time there would be better cures, but if you're drowning, and someone throws you a piece of driftwood, why wait for a life raft?

Right away I scheduled an evaluation with Dr. Sollinger in Wisconsin. As Mom and I sat in his waiting room, I reflected on that day in the doctor's office in London when we had first learned about my diabetes. Bouncing from hope to doubt and back, I wondered if a pancreas transplant would finally right the great wrong of diabetes, or if indeed it would make matters worse.

Dr. Sollinger guided me through my decision. He confirmed that I needed a new kidney and explained that I could get a kidney transplant alone or I could get one simultaneously with a pancreas transplant. A kidney transplant alone would be a simpler operation and easier recovery, but I would need to take immunosuppression drugs to prevent the transplanted kidney from being rejected, *and* I would still be diabetic. Immunosuppression would make diabetes harder to manage and could lead to diabetic kidney disease in the transplanted kidney. Adding a pancreas at the same time as the kidney could extend the life of that new kidney and free me of diabetes. A simultaneous kidney-and-pancreas transplant would be a bigger procedure and more complicated recovery. A higher incidence of surgical complications was associated with kidney-pancreas transplants, but the overall success rate in Wisconsin was 85 percent, and I was certainly an ideal candidate for the bigger operation. As he spoke I noticed on a side table the picture of his children and his family at a ski resort. Mom told me she'd heard that Dr. Sollinger had been a world-class skier. Seeing his jovial face and magnanimous personality, I knew that he understood what life should be, what I wanted *my* life to be. I found myself desperately wanting to be accepted into the program.

"So, Deborah," Dr. Sollinger said, "you must think about this and let me know what you want to do."

I looked directly into his gaze, resisting the urge to just say "yes" without any further reflection. Checking that urge, I said, "I want to go to the transplant floor and speak to some of the patients first if that's okay."

The transplant coordinator took Mom and me to meet a patient, a priest actually, who had received a new pancreas and kidney two months earlier and was back in the hospital trying to stop the immune attack that was causing some rejection.

"You know what?" he said to me with a steady gaze, "Even if I were to lose these organs tomorrow, I would do this again just to have two more months free of diabetes."

After a moment I said. "I can't imagine what it would be like to be free of diabetes. I just can't imagine."

Then a most wrenching and fortuitous thing happened. As Mom and I walked back down the hall toward the nurse's station, talking about how incredible it was to meet someone who had been cured of my "incurable" disease, Mom's attention was caught by the name card on one of the patients' doors we passed. She stopped momentarily to look, but then quickly turned back to me and we continued. When we got to the nurse's station, Mom went to talk to one of the nurses, while I asked another about the recovery time after surgery and what to expect. Then I noticed Mom go back to peek into the room that had caught her attention.

As we walked back to the elevator I asked, "Mom, what were you looking at in that room?"

She thought for a minute and then said, "Well, I wasn't sure if I should say anything to you, but that was my cousin Mac."

I stopped. "What? Your cousin Mac? The diabetic one? Mom, we should go back and visit with him. This can all wait, you know. We're not in that big a rush. I've never met him."

"Sweetie, he's dying. He's blind and on dialysis. They told me he's in and out of a coma. They're not very optimistic about his recovery."

"Can't they give him a new kidney and pancreas? That's what they do here isn't it?"

"He's too far gone. He wouldn't survive the surgery."

After a lifetime without ever meeting, my cousin Mac and I had both ended up in the same hospital in Wisconsin; he to die, and I to be cured. I knew then, with absolute certainty, that I wanted to take my chances with a pancreas transplant rather than end up like Mac. I wanted to wake up each morning knowing that the day ahead could be better than the one before. Something better than pancreas transplants would no doubt come along, but if I was "too far gone," it wouldn't help.

When we got back to Dr. Sollinger's office, I told him, "I want a new kidney and pancreas."

"Then we will get them for you," he replied.

Chapter 7

My Broken Dream

That life is worth living is the most necessary of assumptions,
and were it not assumed, the most impossible of conclusions.
—*George Santayana,* Reason in Common Sense

In the small hours of the morning on April 5, 1993, a
thirty-nine-year-old man died of a brain hemorrhage in
Ohio. His family reached selflessly beyond their grief to
donate the organs and tissues from the lifeless body of the
young man they had loved. It was an act that makes mockery
of war, racism, hatred, and crime, an act that restores faith in
humanity. The pancreas and one kidney were offered to the
University of Wisconsin Hospital, where a sample of my
blood was mixed with the donor's and a match was established. If the organ recovery went smoothly, I would be called
to go to Wisconsin for my transplant.

The next morning I sat in my office with work papers piled

up beside me while I unknowingly became a central figure in the drama taking place hundreds of miles away. A young Japanese broker called from London with concerns about immigration proceedings for his transfer to New York. I had begun to feel shaky and sweaty so, as I spoke on the phone, I pricked my finger to summon the little red messenger bringing a report from within. With more than fifteen thousand practice runs and the aim of an expert marksman, I released the bead of blood onto a tiny circle on the glucose-testing strip. Just then the light on my personal phone line lit up to tell me I had a call. It was Marilyn, the transplant coordinator from Madison, telling me they had organs for me.

"Hang on, Marilyn, I'll be right back," I said and quickly finished my call with the young broker. "Hi, I'm back."

"Deb," she said, "you need to get here as soon as you can. Go ahead and make your travel arrangements and call me back when you have a flight so I can know when to expect you, okay?"

"I'm so excited Marilyn! I'll call you back in a few minutes."

The phone clicked and she was gone. Holding the handset in front of my eyes, I looked at it for a moment in disbelief. Then I was overjoyed. What had seemed like endless months of waiting, of making no long-term plans, for fear of missing "my call," were over. The seasons had changed from spring to summer to fall and back to winter as I had waited. With each new season I carefully packed my bag so I would be ready when the call came, but I hadn't unpacked my winter clothes and already the trees along my street in New York were shimmering with green. I had to hurry. I went to my closet and started throwing clothes onto the bed, a most unusual collection that somehow seemed appropriate at the time. Hastily I wedged them into my suitcase and, with a quick glance around my apartment, closed the door behind me, walking away from my life of needles and restrictions.

Six hours later I underwent surgery. The very next day, pushing a pole carrying little bags of fluid dripping through a tube that had been inserted under my collarbone, I shuffled down the sterile, monochromatic corridor. Mom, who had flown from Bermuda while I was in surgery, was, as always, there to support me. For twenty-three years not a day had passed without injections, diets, and worry about my blood sugar going too high or too low. There I was, twenty-four hours after the surgery, with normal blood-sugar levels—without insulin. I had taken more than twenty-five thousand insulin injections without this natural balance of glucose, insulin, and energy for even a single day. What I remember most about waking up after my transplant was the feeling that, for the first time since I was ten years old, my health, instead of getting progressively worse, could actually improve.

For ten days I was given infusions of a very powerful immunosuppression medication called OKT3 to protect my newly transplanted organs during their period of acclimation. The first few days sent me into sweaty, feverish convulsions, with my temperature climbing to 104°F as I retched and retched. The muscles in my back and neck became rigid, and I shook uncontrollably. The nurse infused Demerol into the small tube. Within minutes I was semiconscious and comfortable. Each day on OKT3 was better than the day before. By the tenth day, confident that my immune system had been suppressed enough to tolerate my transplanted organs, the doctors stopped the medicine. Blood was sent to the lab early every morning for testing, and by late morning a long row of numbers was added to the big yellow chart pinned to a cork-board near my door. Every afternoon a white-coated entourage entered my room to consult the big yellow chart about my progress before asking me for a second opinion. As they talked among themselves they were delighted at their success and at how straightforward my course had been.

It had been only two weeks since my surgery when my discharge papers were summarily signed and last minute details were put in place for an early morning departure. My new kidney purged the excess fluid that had pooled in my limbs, making me feel slim and limber again. The numbers on the wall chart—potassium, phosphorus, creatinine, blood pressure, and blood sugar—were all normal, without medication.

My sister Lesley was getting married in England at the beginning of June, in six weeks. Mom and I looked at pictures of her engagement ring and the airy white dress she had chosen. My childhood dream of being my sister's maid of honor at an English summer wedding was coming true and, as in my childhood dream, I wasn't diabetic. A month's supply of medicine was delivered in a large brown grocery bag to take with me in the morning. That night I lay awake looking at the moon through the hospital window and sobbed with joy and relief that diabetes was over. I thought about my donor, the man who had given me back my health, and wondered what he had dreamed of and hoped for when he looked at the moon. I fell into the exhausted heavy sleep of a soldier resting after the fighting is over and the enemy has retreated.

But as I slept my body became a battlefield, with my newly transplanted organs fighting the vigilant militia of my immune system. The defense that had protected me through childhood diseases, scraped knees, and infections had become my adversary. The new pancreas and kidney were seen as foreign invaders, and my immune system knew only to attack. In the morning I awoke with a fever. Blood was drawn, cultures were taken and then we waited to see if I had an infection or if I was rejecting the organs. If it were rejection, I would need more immunosuppression drugs, but if it were infection those drugs would only make it worse. And so we waited. Mom paced the halls and hovered around the nurses' station waiting for news of what I was up against.

When the numbers came back, they indicated that I was rejecting my new organs. *Please, please* don't let me be diabetic again, I pleaded silently. The doctors converged in discussion and another ten-day round of immunosuppression drugs was prescribed. As before, the medicine made me vomit and go into feverish convulsions; yet my "numbers" rallied and again I believed the obstacles were behind me, that my immune system had accepted my new organs. I was rescheduled for discharge. Then the next morning, as if aroused by my sense of hope, my temperature started to climb defiantly, and I was eye to eye with the fear that had huddled behind my barricade of optimism: the transplant wasn't working. In spite of a three-week regimen of the most powerful and effective immunosuppression drugs available at the time, my body wasn't accepting my new organs.

My doctors were in agreement that I would be at too great a risk of depleting my immune system to a dangerously low level if I were given another round of OKT3, so they decided to try a seven-day course with a milder immunosuppression drug. I braced myself for the familiar feverish convulsions but there were none, only retching. With one particularly violent paroxysm of vomiting, I felt the stitches holding the inside lining of my abdomen pop open like a zipper breaking. With my insides pressing against the fragile purple incision running down the center of my torso, my abdomen ballooned as if I was in my third trimester of pregnancy. Instinctively, Mom pushed the call button and ran for help. In less than a minute she returned with two nurses and a wide, elasticized canvas brace with a Velcro closure to hold me together. A doctor examined the damage and said that it would need to be repaired surgically. There was no imminent danger as long as I was kept bound together, so the operation was deferred until I could recover from the transplant surgery and the large doses of immunosuppression that had left me weak and vulnerable to infection. Lesley's wedding was fast approaching and, in spite of my new pancreas, it seemed that another of life's great moments would pass me by.

The next time my numbers improved there was no time for optimism, because almost immediately they started to reverse. The doctors had only one more weapon in their arsenal to save my new kidney and pancreas—radiotherapy. The days of radiotherapy began when my limp body was lifted onto a gurney and wheeled to the basement of an isolated wing of the hospital. Electronic doors opened automatically and closed behind us as I was pushed down narrow concrete halls to a cold room where I was placed under a cameralike machine reaching down from the ceiling. A red light started flashing, and a siren that sounded like an air raid echoed in the chamber. All of a sudden I was alone. The people who had brought me to that place disappeared while I was left tied to the gurney as the radioactive rays ricocheted through my body.

The radiotherapy worked, and my numbers improved once more. Again I believed the worst was behind me, only to be slapped down by a climbing temperature. The recurring nightmare was relentless. Blood cultures were taken, the central line that had been embedded beneath my collarbone was removed and replaced with a new one, and scans were done. Finally word came back that I had developed a fungal infection. A gurney arrived to wheel me off for yet another procedure. My body was lifted onto a steel table under a large scanner, and small rubber hoses were inserted into my back, abdomen, and side. Bags were attached to the hoses to collect the fungus as it drained. A drug to fight the infection was infused through the tube in my neck. Each day brought the pain of new procedures. My tolerance was eroding fast, yet a small drop of the hope I had arrived with remained. I believed I would walk out of that hospital free of diabetes.

The smallest exertion left me breathless—putting my arm in a sleeve, a slipper on my foot or a stroke of my brush through my thin, lifeless hair—yet every day I got dressed in street clothes. Mom helped me with the seemingly futile task, which began by 8:00 A.M. and took several hours to complete; yet it was by no means a fruitless task. It was an exercise in will and a restatement of my commitment to get well. My hands and arms had become so weak that holding a pen to write left me no energy to form words. Opening a bottle of pills led to tears of frustration. Mom, too, was emotionally and physically exhausted, and I worried about how much more she could take. The days slowed to a crawl. Every morning I was taken to occupational therapy in a wheelchair, feeling humiliated and demoralized as I sat there pushing brightly colored plastic pegs into holes and building houses with wooden screws and bricks. The occupational therapists tried to encourage my feeble progress with comments like, "Oh! That's terrific" and "Wow! You're doing great." Comparatively speaking I suppose I was, but it was a long way to snowskiing hell bent down a black diamond slope or winning a new consulting contract in Europe. I knew it would be a hard climb back to a meaningful life from that small linoleum-floored room where I was challenged to tie shoe laces and thread beads; but I was alive and determined to stay free of diabetes.

Lesley's wedding was drawing near and still my new organs had not settled in; I knew I wouldn't be able to go. When the day finally arrived for Mom to leave for England, I shuffled to the front door of the hospital pushing a wheelchair for balance. Waving goodbye, I smiled for her.

"Bring me lots of pictures and tell Lesley how much I wanted to be with her," I called. Lesley had always been supportive and loving, even when diabetes thrust me onto center stage, focusing all the attention on me. Where other siblings might have been resentful, my sister and brother have been fiercely loyal and protective of me. This was Lesley's day, and I did not want it to be compromised.

Shortly after Mom left, seven weeks after arriving in Madison, I was discharged to a local motel. My excitement was underscored with apprehension. I had grown dependent on the experienced transplant nurses and I felt vulnerable going out on my own with the new regimen of medications. For a fleeting moment I wanted my diabetes back. There were so many pills, I could barely walk, drainage tubes with little plastic bags still hung out of my side, and I was alone. I had never regained enough strength to have my abdomen restitched since it had popped open, so my middle was still tenuously held together with the elastic and Velcro brace.

Less than twenty-four hours after I checked into the motel, my fever returned and I was readmitted to the hospital—defeated and drained of hope. I found some small consolation in learning that a virus called CMV was causing my fever and that it could be treated with intravenous drugs. It would be a ten-day course, but the doctors were optimistic that there would be no further complications. The surgery to mend the ruptured sutures was scheduled for August. Mom was due to return at the same time as the CMV treatment would finish. If everything went well, she would be able to take me home to recuperate. I would return in August to be restitched.

But as the week passed, the fever worsened. My lungs filled with fluid, and I was rushed to an intensive-care room on the transplant floor. The fluid was drained and my breathing eased, but the fever continued unchecked. Unable to eat, drink, go to the bathroom, or walk, I huddled under the blankets with my teeth chattering from chills.

"This is a mystery," the doctors said, shaking their heads.

"There are no mysteries. Keep looking," I beseeched them. There are hundreds of different chemicals, cells, and temperatures in the human body, all being controlled within a precise range. I was sure that when they diverged from that range, there had to be a reason. As the doctors searched for answers from their knowledge and experience, I worked to communicate the things I could "feel" in my body, afraid that the answers would be found too late to affect the outcome. At last, the doctors concluded that I had an abdominal infection, and that by opening me up and "washing out" my abdominal cavity, they could solve the problem.

Surgery was scheduled for June 5, the day of Lesley's wedding. Alone and afraid, I was wheeled into surgery. Tears ran in lines down my face as I stared blankly into the saucerlike lights, surrounded by strangers talking in hushed tones under their face masks and green scrubs. The clinical smell of disinfectant permeated the frigid operating room. In the far reaches of my mind, I could hear wedding bells ringing out across the fields in the south of England. I pictured my sister in her frothy white gown, her coppery red hair adorned with flowers. Her deep blue eyes would be enlivened with love and dreams of starting a family. Her good friend Liz was her bridesmaid, and even though I was in surgery in Madison, she kept me in her heart as her maid of honor.

After the surgery I lay despondent in my hospital bed in Intensive Care and thought about dying. My intellectual perception of death had been replaced by a physical understanding of mortality. In those dark days, dying was as real as living. What would happen if I lived was as much a mystery to me as what would happen if I died. *If I die*, I thought, *there will be no more pain.* Days, minutes, hours, nights, seconds—they were meaningless. Nurses came and went with their cheerful greetings and happy wishes. I smiled back weakly. Staring at the doorway, I willed Mom to return. I wanted to die, but I didn't want to die alone. At some point during the thread of time that wove through my consciousness, Mom came through the door and straight to my side. My voice was small but she listened earnestly as I explained how I wanted to die. Without negating my feelings she agreed that my life, as it was then, was not a life for me.

"Dr. Sollinger is sure you'll get better. You can always die," she said, "but now you have the chance to live." Mom handed me a letter Lesley had given her for me. I was too weak to open it so Mom took the letter out of the envelope and passed it to me. Lesley wrote:

It has been such a strange year with so many good things happening in my life and so many bad ones in yours. More than anything in the world I wanted you here to share this special, special time in my life. You have always been in my thoughts—with every part of choosing the dress, reception, and flowers down to the service we went to at the church and finally the ceremony itself. I kept imagining what you would say about this, or think about that, and all the time it was with a thought of what you would say that I took steps forward. It has always been you who has given me the courage and the humour to get the best out of life—I sometimes almost hear your voice encouraging me when I am frightened or worried. I even felt special in a material way on my wedding day wearing the dress that you bought for me—it was like you were there—it was such a beautiful and whimsical dress that it had a personality of its own. You will never know how much I missed and needed having you there. Well, there has to be a dream coming true for you soon. . . ."

The letter was so full of her love and wisdom that it beckoned me to find the value of my life beyond mere existence. Without knowing the ambushes that lay ahead on my journey to an insulin-free life, I made a silent pact to keep my focus on the ultimate goal—freedom from diabetes. Yet only two days later I was overcome with fatigue and thirst and my legs turned thick with fluid. With a deep sense of foreboding, I asked the nurse to test my blood sugar. The diabetic ritual seemed unfamiliar as I anxiously waited for the number on the monitor as it counted down forty-five seconds.

"My blood sugar feels high," I choked. It couldn't be. It had to be a reaction caused by one of the medications. I couldn't look at the monitor. Maybe if I didn't look, everything would be all right. When the monitor beeped, I looked. "It's four-sixty!" I screamed, "Call Dr. Sollinger. Please hurry! Get me some insulin! Quickly! Maybe we can fix it!" I urged. My heart raced. I felt sick.

The nurse reappeared holding a syringe half full of insulin and asked, "Do you want to do this or should I?"

"You do it. I'm not sure I remember how!"

"Dr. Sollinger was called, and he wants you to go right away for a scan. He'll meet you down there when it's done."

The gurney, my hospital limousine, arrived and whisked me down to Nuclear Medicine. I slid under the all-seeing eye of the large metal structure and felt the cold dye flow into my arm. Drowsiness overcame me, and I drifted into a deep sleep. I was awakened by the voice of the technician telling me the scan was finished. Had it been a nightmare that my blood sugar was high? Or had something really gone wrong? I was wheeled out into the hallway. Dr. Sollinger had his hand on Mom's shoulder and when she turned to me, there were tears in her eyes. She couldn't speak. My cheerful, vibrant Dr. Sollinger looked at me sadly. "Deb, the organs have rejected."

Anger, desperation, disbelief, and grief surged to the surface. The feelings were too big to let in. I closed my eyes and forced them back into the inner space where the beast of diabetes resided. The fight was over. I floated on the tranquility of resignation that follows unfathomable disappointment.

My new organs were removed on June 12, but because my native kidney and pancreas had been left in place, I had those old, damaged organs to keep me going. Thirty-five people had come to Madison for kidney-pancreas transplants since I was admitted on April 6. All but two of us left, free of diabetes. My diabetes returned with full force with my blood sugar fluctuating as wildly as it had before the transplant. Cycles of nausea, thirst, and sweaty headaches returned. I went back to my four to eight daily injections of insulin and blood tests, along with Epoiten injections to fight anemia, blood-pressure monitoring, and diuretics. My left leg had swelled to twice its normal size; between that and the anemia I couldn't walk more than five yards. I knew it was time to leave the hospital: there had been too many procedures, too many operations and too many disappointments. The doctors and nurses had done all they could for me.

I was discharged over the Fourth of July weekend. It was almost three months since I'd arrived in Madison with such great hope for my future. Mom packed the car and, with my foot up on the dashboard and the passenger seat reclined, we set out to meet my stepfather, Norman, in Wyoming. Mom's flawless determination to right the great wrongs of all my years with diabetes, and my beautiful dream of a life free of diabetes, had amounted to this. We followed a map that would take us to the Grand Teton Mountains without knowing where I would go after that, or why.

Chapter 8

The Road Back

If you can make one heap of all your winnings
And risk it on one turn of pitch and toss,
And lose, and start again at your beginnings
And never breathe a word about your loss;
If you can force your heart and nerve and sinew
To serve your turn long after they are gone
And so hold on when there is nothing in you
Except the Will which says to them: "Hold on!"
—*Rudyard Kipling,* "If"

The highway led us away from Madison. I kept my eyes fixed on the road ahead without looking back. We tracked west through Minnesota, South Dakota, and most of the way across the state of Wyoming. A little spark of joy flickered in the shadow of my disappointment. The air smelled fresh, the dirt looked clean, and I felt better just by being away from the sterile impersonal hospital. The fresh air, open space, and the road stretching out ahead refreshed me, like the first exquisite indulgence after a long fast. I surveyed the scenes rolling past the big, green Buick as we drove twelve hundred miles back to the small summer home Mom and Norman had built in a valley just east of the Grand Teton Mountains.

Mom and I had a carefree three days driving across the Midwest, relieved that, for better or worse, my transplant ordeal was over. After cycling through alternating high-flying hope and plunging despair, I found solace in the steady ache of grief. My left leg stayed turgid with edema. My shoes, leg braces, and jeans didn't fit. I wore sweat pants and a huge slipper and kept my leg raised as much as I could, hoping that the fluid would subside. Once again, food collected in my stomach and became an acidic, undigested mass that made me vomit. The familiar routine of glucose monitoring, insulin injections, and stopping for meals when my blood sugar demanded was no easier or more effective than it had ever been.

Over the next few days, I gazed up at the grandeur of the Tetons and wrestled with decisions about work, my health, and what I should do next. I knew that I could not, would not, go on as a diabetic. I started to make a plan. I'd stay with Mom and Norman in Wyoming until I felt strong enough to return to New York City and my apartment. As soon as I got home, I would find work. It would be a year before I'd be strong enough to go through another transplant, but knowing that the waiting list for organs was long, and that my kidneys wouldn't last much longer, I'd write to Dr. Sollinger to ask to be relisted right away. After ten days of sleeping, eating, and walking as far as I could in the mountain air, I was well on the road to recovery. My heart was in it.

I returned to New York twenty-five pounds lighter than when I'd left and hungry to continue my life somewhere familiar, with people I knew and everyday problems that I could solve. I welcomed back the *weltschmerz* of my days. My small apartment seemed luxurious in contrast to the habitual hospital rooms. It was full of color and soft things. There was no emergency resuscitation equipment poised expectantly on the wall, and no smell of human waste. Most of all, I basked in the privacy and my liberation from the intrusion of the sharp tools of medicine. When people in my neighborhood asked me where I had been, I said either that I'd taken some time off or had been away. It wasn't important for anyone to know. Even if I told them I'd been to Wisconsin for a kidney and pancreas transplant, no words could explain the complicated journey my soul had taken. Few would understand the chance I had taken to be free of a disease that society dismisses as a life-style. My transplant memories were, for now, best forgotten.

I had been restitched in the middle after the organs were removed, my hair had filled in, and I looked presentable, albeit frail. While I was away I had paid my mortgage in New York with checks that had trickled in on outstanding receivables from my consulting practice, but my money was almost gone. I needed to find some income, and fast. Ideally I wanted to resume my consulting work from home because I was still plagued by persistent nausea, fatigue, neuropathy, anemia, edema, and, of course, diabetes.

When I was in the hospital in Madison, Tom, one of my colleagues from New York, had rerouted his return trip from a business trip to Chicago so that he could pay me a surprise visit. I remembered the look of shock that spread across his face when he saw me. We had spoken several times on the telephone and I had asked about work as if it were my biggest concern. When he asked when I'd be back, I had answered, "I've had a few little setbacks, but I'll be back at work soon." It wasn't until he showed up at the hospital that he understood I'd known too much pain and was near the end of my endurance. My hair was sparse and brittle, my face gaunt and colorless. I struggled to support my swollen and stapled middle on spindly legs. I was wearing a maternity dress and sneakers as he pushed my wheelchair out into the sun. His being there gave me a visceral sense of my inadequacy and of the life that I couldn't reach—and I could see that he wanted to get away from my sickness. As he left I had wanted to say, "I'll be back soon," but that would have sounded absurd coming from my pathetic form. His goodbyes had an ambiguous finality.

Recalling this incident I had to acknowledge that if my clients knew how truly fragile my health was, I wouldn't be hired on a bet. Working from home, where I could conceal the worst of it, was my only recourse. So like an ingenue preparing for one more performance in a long-running play, I donned my customary mask of well-being and went down to Wall Street to solicit an assignment from one of my former clients. My client worked with Tom and had heard I'd had a failed organ transplant, but I was sure he didn't know the full extent of my ongoing diabetes. My charade paid off with an assignment to coordinate and write a strategic plan for the company's group of brokerage, information, and technology subsidiaries.

I was given an office in the firm's Water Street headquarters to use whenever I needed to meet people downtown. If it hadn't been for that office I'm not sure how I would have managed the numerous meetings that would otherwise have required walking from location to location. On days when I was at my weakest, I'd consolidate my thoughts and draft the strategic document at home.

At home I worked in an old pair of shorts and socks, but to go downtown I had to look professional. It was August in New York and the air was thick with steamy heat. My leg braces were intolerably hot and my swollen legs so frozen by neuropathy that I could barely walk. Standing without losing my balance was impossible. The long skirts I wore to hide my braces, and the lace-up ankle boots that stayed tied to my numb feet, left me feeling clumsy and frumpy around the other women in their stylish suits with short, pencil-thin skirts and feminine shoes. My lack of style embarrassed me and wiped away my confidence. After work the young brokers would go out to bars and restaurants. I'd work until everyone had left for the evening so my colleagues wouldn't see me stumble out. I couldn't negotiate the stairs in the subways or even the steps up into a bus, so I took taxis to and from work. At the end of the day, exhausted, I'd test my blood sugar, take insulin, eat, and fall into bed.

Six months had passed since I left Wisconsin and I was ready to try another kidney and pancreas transplant. Sitting at my desk, I took out a pad of paper and wrote a letter to Dr. Sollinger. The reply was swift, warm, and inconclusive. The letter ended with Dr. Sollinger's assurance that he would give another simultaneous kidney and pancreas transplant "a good second chance," but the middle paragraphs had none of the optimism and confidence that had won my trust sixteen months earlier. "The best time for transplantation," he wrote, "will most likely be the time when your kidney function starts to deteriorate in a significant way. At that time you will have to make a choice between a kidney transplant alone or a kidney-pancreas transplant." *What?* A kidney transplant *alone?* What was he saying? I was heading into the crippling stages of late-afternoon diabetes, and there wasn't a doctor out there who would tell me that insulin therapy would stop its progression. Getting a pancreas in addition to a kidney would reinstate absolutely normal blood-sugar levels. I *had* to get a pancreas, didn't I?

"The best we can do," the letter continued, "is to make sure that the organs are extremely well matched. We have done this a few times in the past for re-transplants, and it usually seems to work." When I had first met Dr. Sollinger, his conversation had been punctuated with phrases like "Don't worry, we have lots of experience in this" and "You'll do fine." Now I sensed reserve and caution. Why would I forego a new pancreas and the chance to be free of the disease that was surely disabling me? Whether I wanted a kidney-pancreas, or kidney transplant alone, the letter had said I should wait until my kidneys deteriorated further. I let the letter fall to the floor as the realization hit me that maybe, after all, I would end up on dialysis—that waiting room where I would linger until a door would open to either a kidney transplant or death. Within two years half of all diabetics on dialysis die from heart and vascular disease, infection, or suicide. A new pancreas was my only chance to improve my health. Yet my failed attempt the first time had left me graphically aware of the surgical risk and morbidity that could follow the double organ transplant. I wondered if, maybe, instead of getting both a kidney and a pancreas, I *should* opt for the easier procedure of a kidney transplant alone? But then I would still have diabetes *and* I would have to take immunosuppression drugs to prevent the kidney from being rejected. And there would be nothing to stop diabetic kidney disease from attacking a new kidney. My secondary diabetic complications were progressing too quickly, and diabetes research was moving too slowly, to produce safer ways to be cured in time. I picked the letter up from the floor as tears dripped off my face. My dream of being cured was being slowly eclipsed.

Feeling trapped, I fell into a dark depression. Diabetes was killing me, but a pancreas transplant might be too dangerous to try again. Somebody, somewhere must have been in my situation before. What did they do? How did it work out? I couldn't be the only person who had ever wanted to have another kidney-pancreas transplant after a failed attempt. Perhaps I was giving up too easily. Gradually a new resolve started to flicker and I called my doctor in New York to ask if he could introduce me to other people in my position. He told me about an upcoming lecture at New York Hospital by Dr. David Sutherland, a world-renowned expert in the field of pancreas transplantation. My doctor said that several of his patients who already had, or were waiting to have, transplants would be there, and that if I could go, he would introduce me to them.

New York Hospital was only two blocks from my apartment, but because of my neuropathy I allowed a full thirty minutes to walk to the lecture. I was one of the first to get there and chose a chair near some other early arrivals. My doctor came over to introduce me to one of his patients, Fran, a bubbly, friendly young woman with a great sense of humor. Fran was the all-American picture of health. I was disappointed at first because I had hoped to meet a transplant candidate or recipient, but by the time the lecture began, I realized I had—Fran was on Dr. Sutherland's kidney-pancreas waiting list at the University of Minnesota. I knew she understood the part of my life I'd hidden for so long. She too had perfected the diabetic art of looking healthy on the outside while the inside crumbled. Fran was in her mid-twenties and had been diabetic since she was seven. She was just starting dialysis.

After the lecture, our doctor introduced us to others of his patients who were pancreas transplant recipients. We asked them dozens of questions. When it was time to leave Fran and I shared a taxi, and she dropped me off at my apartment on her way home. We talked on the phone often during the following weeks, sharing our fears and our dreams of being cured. She was wise beyond her years, with an endearing blend of insight into the horror of diabetes and an irrepressible joie de vivre. Often we spoke of diabetic experiences that we didn't need to explain, because both of us already knew. Our conversations always circled back to pancreas transplants.

We decided to organize a picnic for the pancreas recipients we had met at the lecture. I talked one of my client companies into donating their boat to take us for a three-hour cruise around Manhattan. Fran and I called the seven people on our list to invite them to come, and we arranged sandwiches, fruit, and drinks. It was a beautiful summer day. Everyone we invited came. Mike had just returned from having a kidney-pancreas transplant. Mitchel had been free of diabetes for eight years since his kidney-pancreas transplant. Susan had gone blind when she was twenty but finally was free of diabetes after several transplants: a kidney alone that had failed, a kidney-pancreas that had failed, and then another kidney-pancreas transplant that worked perfectly. Greg had just returned from a hundred-mile bicycle race.

He'd had his kidney-pancreas transplant three years earlier without a day of trouble since. Then there was Bob, the quintessential Nice Guy in his blue jeans and denim shirt.

Bob was a California-born, forty-something investment manager. Based in London, he relished the excitement of living in Europe. You couldn't help but like Bob because he liked you. Tall, unpretentious, and fun loving, he had an unthreatening intelligence that made people want to know more about him. He'd never been sick a day in his life, except for diabetes. But when he went home to California to celebrate the Fourth of July a year earlier, his life had started to unravel; in less than a year he was on dialysis. His precipitous slide began when the backs of his eyes hemorrhaged. His doctors drained out the blood and filled the void with a clear fluid so he could see. Next he underwent coronary bypass surgery to repair the damage to his heart caused by diabetes. Then his kidneys failed, and he was added to the kidney-and-pancreas transplant waiting list. In spite of all he had been through, the idea of a transplant scared him most. He was going to go home to California to wait for his call that a donor had been found. The bonds I formed that day were the genesis of what would later become the Insulin-Free World Foundation.

Fran asked me if I wanted to go with her to her dialysis classes where she was learning peritoneal dialysis, a system that could be done at home on a continuous basis instead of in three-hour intervals, three times a week, at the hospital. So I went with her and watched as she dripped bags of cleansing solution through a tube that had been surgically implanted in her belly. Fran's determined optimism didn't belong in that place with its scuffed linoleum floor and antiseptic smell. It was summer, and she should have been roller-blading in Central Park, not learning how to turn the clamps on her dialysis tubing and groaning as cramping pain clawed its way along her abdominal wall. When her belly was filled she allowed the fluid, heavy with her metabolic waste, to flow out into a deflated plastic bag on the floor. From time to time she weighed the bag of cloudy water to calculate how much remained inside her. When all the fluid had flowed out, she closed off the clamps on the tubing, so she could refill her abdomen with fresh fluid. Her abdomen stayed filled with that fluid for three hours, then the ritual would begin again.

I was with Fran when her dialysis supplies were delivered to her tiny, one-bedroom apartment, opposite the American Museum of Natural History. The boxes overwhelmed the small space; dialysis had taken over her body, her schedule, and her home. We checked the items in the boxes against the packing list; tape, clamps, scales, IV pole, alcohol, tubing, face masks, sterile gloves, and bags and bags of fluid. I was more convinced than ever that dialysis is a limbo where people wait for transplants and the chance to go back to living, or slip into death. The clock was already ticking for Fran. I cried for her, and I cried for myself, because my kidneys were deteriorating as hers had and soon I would be living a life like hers.

While Fran was caught in the trappings of dialysis and diabetes, I got a call from Bob's mother in California; he had died from gastrointestinal complications of diabetes. Although I hadn't known him well, Bob's death affected me deeply. Only eighteen months earlier he had been a "healthy diabetic." Now he was dead. There had been three of us on the boat who hadn't received new pancreases—Fran was on dialysis, Bob was dead, and there was me.

My brother, who was at that time selling MRI software to hospitals, called excitedly to give me the name of a pancreas transplant surgeon he'd heard about in Minnesota. Dr. David Sutherland, he said, was one of the pioneers of pancreas transplantation, and the University of Minnesota had the world's oldest and largest pancreas transplant program. What was more, Dr. Sutherland did pancreas transplants alone, pancreas transplants after kidney transplants, pancreas transplants from living donors, and *retransplants*. Dr. Sutherland. The name caught my attention, because most of the people on our boat trip had been transplanted by Dr. Sutherland. He was the speaker at the lecture where Fran and I first met, and he was Fran's transplant surgeon too. I took down his telephone number and as soon as I said good-bye to Blair, I dialed. Within a minute, I was speaking directly to Dr. Sutherland. I explained my situation and he told me to make an appointment to come to the transplant center at the University of Minnesota Hospital for an evaluation. Half afraid of what would happen if I was accepted for a pancreas transplant, and half afraid of what would happen if I wasn't, I flew to Minneapolis to see him.

Dr. Sutherland had scrutinized my medical history and the charts that I had sent him. After two days of tests to make sure I was well enough to sustain another transplant surgery, he told me, in his confident, understated way, that my chance of succeeding was "good." Hope and joy charged through me. I wanted to turn somersaults, knowing that I would have a chance to try again.

Chapter 9

Diabetes' Last Stand

Imagine a world in which people thought diabetes had already been cured. They thought insulin was a cure and that our children would be just fine.

— *Juvenile Diabetes Foundation International*

One Monday in the summer of 1994, the heat in New York hovered at ninety-five degrees for the third day in a row. The clammy humidity clung to my skin. It had been almost twenty-four hours since food or fluids had stayed in my rebellious stomach and I was sure my kidneys had finally given up the fight allowing poisonous toxins to accumulate in my body. I called my doctor only to learn from his office manager that he was away until the following day. She told me to go straight to the emergency room at New York University Hospital and page a Dr. Levine. She would be expecting me. Any frequent patron of medical services in New York City knows

that the last place on earth you want to go when you're sick
is to an emergency room. Something was very wrong with
me, though, so without giving it another thought, I caught
a cab and went right over. I told the person at registration
that Dr. Levine was expecting me.

"Nobody sees anyone here without going through triage,"
she said flatly.

"But I was told to ask for Dr. Levine to be paged as soon
as I arrived."

"I said nobody sees anyone without going through triage.
Sign the register over there and I'll call when it's your turn." I
signed the register and went to the pay phone to ask my doctor's office please to page Dr. Levine and tell her I was in the
waiting area. Ways to escape from that hostile room with its
security policeman and militant clerks circled through my
head, but I needed help; I had waited too long already. Anyway, I was used to spending hours in the waiting rooms of
doctors' offices and hospitals, where they know you need
them more than they need you. I took a seat. Reaching into
my handbag, I pulled out the plastic bag I kept there for
times when I was sick in taxis or out of reach of a rest room.
Holding the bag open in front of me, I threw up. A man who
was bleeding profusely was wheeled in on a gurney and the
emergency medical service nurse informed the policeman
guarding the door that the man had been shot. I threw up
again. I had waited an hour and a half when an overworked,
underpaid nurse with an "I'm just doing my job attitude"
called my name and said "Sit" as she pointed to the chair by
the desk. Looking down at the forms on her desk, without
making eye contact with me, she asked, "What are you here
for?"

"I haven't been able to keep any food or water down for a day. I'm diabetic and I feel terrible. I was supposed to meet Dr. Levine here."

"Any medical history I should know about other than the diabetes?" she questioned, as if diabetes was an incidental condition that could be described by checking off the little box on her form.

"I had a kidney and pancreas transplant last year, the organs rejected and were removed. I'm waiting for another kidney and pancreas. I'm worried that the nausea may be a worsening of my kidney disease."

"They don't do pancreas transplants," she said as she eyed me skeptically. She checked my temperature and blood pressure, then took me back to a cubicle in the emergency room and had me lie down on a gurney to wait again. Another thirty minutes passed before a nurse came in to draw some blood for testing and put an intravenous access in my arm.

"Dr. Levine is expecting me. Would you page her for me, please?"

"You will be seen by the doctor on call here in the emergency room first. He will coordinate your care." The nurse left the room, leaving me to wait once more.

The indifferent and often irrational bureaucracy that defines the administration of health care was not new to me. I was reminded of my encounter in the patient accounts department several months earlier, shortly after Dr. Sutherland had accepted me into his transplant program. The hospital couldn't add my name to the organ donor waiting list until they'd received assurance that payment would be forthcoming, so I had made an appointment to speak to a patient accounts representative. Because my independent Blue

Cross/Blue Shield policy had covered my first transplant without too much difficulty, I was certain there would be no problem. When my name was called, I went into the little office. I hadn't gotten a word out when the innocuous-looking administrator slammed the door on my dream.

"I'm afraid your insurance won't cover a pancreas transplant," he said apologetically. "Do you have any other means?"

"Uh," I paused, stunned by what he had said. "I have the same policy that I had for the first transplant. There must be some mistake."

"Well, we've got Medicare listed as your primary insurance. Medicare only provides benefits for kidney, liver, lung, and heart transplants, not pancreas transplants."

"I neither want, nor need, to be on Medicare! I've paid high premiums for ten years with Blue Cross/Blue Shield, and I even have a backup policy for things like this," I reasoned, trying to stop the bureaucracy from hacking away at my cure.

"Your Blue Cross/Blue Shield policy is an individual policy. Medicare became your primary insurance when you had your kidney transplant."

"How can they do that? Surely I have a say in what insurance I buy? I didn't ask for the government's help. I don't need it. I'm not on dialysis. In fact, I don't even have a kidney transplant because it was removed! I don't qualify for Medicare!" I protested.

"I'm sorry," the man said, shaking his head.

I had returned to New York utterly disillusioned. I had come too far to be stopped by bureaucracy. There *had* to be a way. What would it say on my tombstone? "She died from bad insurance?" In desperation I took out a home equity loan of sixty thousand dollars to put on deposit at the hospital so I could once again be added to the organ waiting list. Medicare had overridden the insurance I had worked so hard to protect for more than a decade. When I was at my sickest, Medicare had necessitated my going further into debt. Something was terribly wrong with the system.

I looked at my watch. It was four o'clock. Three hours had passed since I'd arrived at the hospital and I was still in the emergency room waiting to see a doctor. People could die waiting in the emergency room, I thought cynically. I sighed and yawned and wondered if I should go home and wait to see my own doctor in the morning. Still the nausea was coming in waves and I kept retching into the bedpan. Forty-five minutes later a young, imperious doctor strode in and dutifully completed the rote list of medical history questions.

"Ms. Butterfield, we'll need to keep you here until we have your blood results. Do you have any questions?" he asked as he turned to leave.

"I need to check my blood-sugar level and I don't have my monitor here. I'll probably need some insulin too."

"Just be patient, we'll get to that when we have your blood work back."

"I've waited three hours and nothing has been done. Dr. Levine is expecting me and is familiar with my history. I've asked several times to speak to her and. . . ."

"She left half an hour ago."

"When will she be back?"

"In the morning," he said without a hint of regret.

How will I ever make it through the night in here, I thought? My medicines were at home and I needed to be able to test my blood sugar often, take insulin as needed, and drink lots of fluids. This was not going to work. I had been living in my diabetic body for 24 hours a day, 365 days a year, for 24 years. That was 210,240 hours. If I had worked that many hours in a 40-hour-per-week job, I would have 106 years of experience. Yet, as was often the case, the doctor dismissed me as a layperson and assumed power of attorney over my decisions. It was a typical example of a chronic illness being cared for in a medical system designed to take care of short-term illness and trauma. In an acute-care system, doctors make decisions about diagnosis, treatment, and rehabilitation with minimal consultation with the patient. But diabetes is chronic, and people who live with diabetes are required to be experts in their own care. Young doctors, trying to exercise their newly acquired knowledge, often have a hard time including the experience of their patients in the equation. Too tired to be angry, too weak for frustration, I stated calmly, "I'd like to be discharged now. I'll come back in the morning."

"To discharge you now and readmit you in the morning causes a great deal of paperwork. And you would be leaving against my advice."

"I understand and appreciate your concern. I'll be at my home telephone number. Please will you notify me of any extraordinary lab findings from my blood work?" And I left.

The next morning I was feeling much better. The hospital never called me so I went down to my office on Water Street assuming that my blood tests must have been unremarkable. I was in and out of meetings from the time I arrived at work until four-thirty, when I returned to my office to check my calls. Predictably, the light on my telephone was flashing. The first message got my attention.

"Ms. Butterfield, this is New York University Hospital. Please call us immediately." The caller left a number.

I stared at the phone, reluctant to make the call. This would be dialysis. This was what I had dreaded. The threat that had stalked me for several years was here. I would have to go to the hospital three times a week for three hours. I was to be dependent on a machine after all. No donor had been found in time. Maybe matching organs would never be found. I had developed so many antibodies (protein molecules that are part of the immune system's defense against foreign tissue) from my transplant in Madison that only 16 percent of the Type B blood donors would be compatible, and only 8 percent of the population nationwide has Type B blood. Not all people who die can be donors; they must be brain dead so the organs are still functioning when they are recovered. My father, with his trademark boundless love, and without a moment's hesitation, had offered me one of his kidneys, only to be disqualified by ill health. It was a crap shoot and I had lost. I picked up the receiver and pressed the numbers on the phone. It rang five times before a voice answered, "Emergency."

"This is Deborah Butterfield returning your call."

"Butterfield? Yes, here you are. Butterfield. You need to come back to the hospital right away. You had a heart attack."

I sat down. "I think there is a mistake. I couldn't have had a heart attack; I'm only thirty-four years old. There is nothing wrong with my heart," I argued.

"The doctor left orders for you to come here right away."

Puzzled and alarmed, I called my doctor's office and was transferred through to him immediately.

"I went to the hospital yesterday and they called me just now to say I had a heart attack!" My voice started to crack. "But I didn't feel anything. How can—"

"Deb, this is not unusual for people with diabetes. Quite often people who have neuropathy like you do don't feel the chest pains associated with a heart attack," he explained. "Try to relax. I've notified the cardiologist at the hospital that you will be coming into the emergency room."

"I'm not going there again! It's a war zone."

"Deb, we need to admit you but there are no beds available in the main hospital. Our best bet is to bring you in through emergency. I'll meet you there. Is there someone we can call for you? Someone who could meet us there?"

I paused. No one in my family lived in New York. Who could understand this surreal situation, I wondered? I gave them Tom's name, Tom Wendel. He had seen this part of me when he visited me in the hospital in Madison, and since then we had become friends. He would know how to reach my mother, who would be at home in Bermuda with Norman, waiting for a phone call from England to tell her that my sister Lesley, who was nine months pregnant, had delivered her first child.

Fifteen minutes later I arrived at the emergency room and this time, with my doctor in tow, I was taken right in. Tom arrived shortly after but wasn't permitted to see me until visiting hours, which lasted for ten minutes only, every hour on the hour. When he finally got to me, his eyes were anxious but his posture strong. He looked suntanned and so out of place. Once again stripped of my dignity, I lay in a short hospital gown with my scarred, skinny legs, in braces and boots, stretched out on the sheets. Nitroglycerin patches and monitors were stuck all over my arms and chest.

"I'm fine, really. This is all a precaution," I told Tom. "They just need to check out abnormal heart enzyme results. Please don't worry." Silently I feared that this was a death sentence. A donor hadn't come in time and now I'd had a heart attack. I thought I wouldn't be eligible for a transplant after all. The diabetes would have its chance to dismember me, one organ, one system, one limb at a time.

"I'm not worried," he said too quickly, and his eyes filled with water. He wanted to help but didn't know how. He held my hand and told me he had talked to Mom and that she would be coming to New York on the next flight out. And he told me that I was an aunt; my sister had a healthy little boy named Harry. Visiting time passed quickly and Tom had to leave. I spent the next forty-five hours lying on a stretcher in the emergency room. Tom came often. There were no windows. I had no sense of day or night. Nothing was familiar. I would watch the doors waiting for Tom's visits. Stretchers were lined up side by side with no more than six inches between them. There was no privacy and no rest. On either side of me were men who had suffered heart attacks in the heat too. People moaned and called for the nurses, but the nurses ignored them. There was no place to wash, only one bathroom, and nothing but crackers and broth to eat. My insulin came late and in the wrong doses. The hospital was full. Those of us in the emergency room had no choice but to wait for beds. Sometime toward the end of those long hours in the emergency room, Tom walked through the doors with Mom. Just as she had been on Lesley's wedding day when I was in surgery in Madison, Mom had been torn between being with Lesley to celebrate a milestone in her life, or being with me to fend off death. Again visiting time passed far too soon, and the nurse came to tell them to leave. Mom started to argue but Tom took her arm and said, "Sara, they don't make exceptions, I already tried that."

Finally, a man in white with a badge that said Transport arrived and pushed my stretcher to an intensive-care room on the cardiac floor. There were four beds and a desk over to one side where a nurse was stationed twenty-four hours a day. The other patients in the suite all had gray hair and gray skin hanging loosely on their bones. There we were—two old men, one old woman, and me—wired to monitors that told the secrets of our heartbeats. The relevance of age must be in how far you are from dying, not how far you are from being born; and if that is so then I surely felt among peers in that cardiac intensive-care unit.

It was a relief to be in a place where Tom and Mom could come and go. Mom stayed in my apartment Thursday night and came and sat all day with me on Friday. Tom, so vital and confident in his dark suit, stopped by on his way to a lunch meeting in midtown. On Friday evening he visited again and this time brought a brown paper bag with a bagel and cream cheese for me and a selection of salads and sandwiches for Mom and him. In a short time he had become quite expert at knowing what worked with my low-potassium, low-phosphorus, low-protein, low-sodium, high-fat, and controlled-carbohydrate diet. We went down to the sitting area and ate at a coffee table overlooking the boat harbor on the East River. For a while I could forget where I was, and why I was there. Half an hour after Mom and Tom left for the evening, Tom called from his apartment.

"This is the IRS and I'm looking for the little old lady with the broken heart," he said with a comical accent.

"You'd better find a younger woman while you've got a chance!" I laughed. I loved the way he sensed my unspoken fears and was open with me about them. He walked through my walls of words and smiles and made friends with the "me" that I hid from the casual observer. Tom was born a generation before me in Jamestown, North Dakota, and in spite of rising to a high-powered position on Wall Street he was endowed with an all-American, proud-to-be-a-marine, take-care-of-Mom charm. In any other time, any other place, I would have loved Tom as a woman loves a man. Perhaps I already did, but the notion of such a powerful and energetic man feeling anything other than pity for me seemed farcical. As I sat in my hospital bed amid the tentacles of the heart monitor and its clammy little pads stuck to my chest, I looked out over the bridges on the East River and told myself that no man could love a woman who had as many problems as I did then. I wiped away tears of loneliness that began to slide down my cheeks. The fading sun of that summer Friday night retreated behind the skyline of New York without so much as an apology.

Very early the next morning I was jarred awake by the telephone ringing next to my bed. I reached through the intravenous tubes and wires attached to the heart monitor and picked up the receiver. "Hello?" I said, trying to sound like the phone hadn't woken me up.

"Hi, Deb, this is Dr. Sutherland."

"Hi! It's so nice of you to call! Did my doctor tell you I was here?"

"No, I just called your apartment and talked to your mom. She told me. Deb, I have a donor for you."

"Oh no! What irony. It's too late, I had a heart attack last week." I heard a pause on the other end. "Dr. Sutherland, what's going to happen to me?"

"Have you had an angiogram?"

"No, but I'm scheduled for one on Monday."

"Can you get one now?"

"They don't move that fast here."

"You could come here for one if they'll let you fly. If the results are good, we could do the transplant afterward. You would be taking a risk though, because if the results aren't favorable, you would have flown all the way out for nothing."

"You mean I wouldn't be eligible?"

"Sometimes we have to do a bypass or some other tune-up on the heart before a patient can go through a transplant safely."

"But you could do it?"

"Deb, we're going to get you through all this. Do you want to try for the donor I just received?"

"Sure I do! I'll call you back once I've figured out how to get there."

I rang the number in my apartment and Mom answered before the first ring was completed. "What did you decide to do?" she asked anxiously.

"I'm going to go for it. Can you come?"

"Yes, of course! I'll pack your suitcase and come over to the hospital."

I rang for the nurse and explained what was happening and that I needed to be discharged immediately. She called the cardiologist and he arrived in less than a minute.

"You shouldn't be traveling," he said with concern. "We don't even know yet what's going on with your heart. At least you certainly shouldn't fly commercially. Could you charter a plane?"

"I'll find a way. I've got to try because the chances of getting a matching donor are against me." And I thought, *There goes more money I haven't earned yet.*

"I'll fill out your discharge papers while you get organized."

"Could you ask someone to disconnect me from all these wires?"

"No problem," he said as he headed for the door. "Oh, and Deb?"

"Yes?"

"I wish you all the best."

The telephone numbers for the charter plane, taxi, transplant floor, and Dr. Sutherland were written on a sticker I had put on my beeper. A nurse disconnected me from the tubes and wires while I arranged for the plane and a taxi. I still knew the routine from the year before when I had gone to Madison for my first transplant. I hoped that this time I wouldn't go through the same desperate struggle with infection and rejection, yet I was committed to taking all the risks again if it gave me the chance to be free of diabetes. I didn't want another transplant, but I couldn't go on being diabetic. At thirty-four years old, I had withstood a heart attack, flirted with kidney failure and vision loss, was paralyzed below my knees, and walked haltingly with braces. There were no guarantees that a new pancreas would stop my decline, but without one my decline was certain.

I woke Tom up next. He sounded foggy but was instantly alert at the news. He listened intently as I explained the plan.

"I'll come over to the hospital right away to see you off. Oh, and Deb? I'll take care of the plane for now."

Tom had been an emphatic and loyal friend throughout my transplant ordeal, and I quietly accepted his support.

"How can I ever thank you? You're a guardian angel."

Chapter 10

My Cure

Gaze into the sky on a starry night and you will see a few thousand stars, most straddling the darkness in a great swath we call the Milky Way. This is all the ancients knew of the universe. Gradually, as telescopes of greater and greater size and resolution have been developed, a universe of unimagined vastness has swum into view.

—*John D. Barrow,* The Origin of the Universe

"Breathe, Deborah, breathe." Monitors were beeping. Tubes were everywhere. I could hear Mom. She was there. As if she had heard my thoughts, she held my hand and said, "Sweetie, I'm here." I opened my eyes for a few seconds and smiled before falling back into a drugged sleep. Twenty-four hours later I was walking and I wasn't taking insulin. A few days after that, I was eating whatever and whenever I wanted.

"My blood sugars are normal," I told Tom on the phone. "Without insulin, they're normal, not just 'in control'—normal! I can eat anything, anytime. I can skip meals if I want."

"What did you have for breakfast?" he asked, wanting to

hear the happiness in my voice as I recounted the joy of eating a normal breakfast.

"Orange juice and a big, sticky cinnamon bun!"

"That's a lot of potassium and carbohydrate, isn't it?"

"Yes," I laughed.

"What's your blood sugar?"

"Eighty-five."

"Terrific!"

No insulin, no blood-glucose tests, no diets, no blood-pressure medicine, no digestion pills—yet every system in my body functioned normally for the first time in years. But this was how it had started in Madison too, and I was anxious. Every day I waited for the wall chart to quantify that my new organs were doing well. And every day they were, until the third week when, with my heart in my throat, I fought off an episode of rejection. But when I returned to New York in the middle of September, everything was stable. My world was no longer marred by diabetes. Events, no matter how familiar, seemed new. At Thanksgiving I walked through the autumn leaves in Central Park and, for the first time since I was ten, ate Thanksgiving dinner with abandon. Gone was the inexplicable embarrassment I had felt at being diabetic. Being a former diabetic and knowing that each day my health could be better than the day before gave me a sense of winning in place of the irrational sense of failure that had accompanied diabetes.

Five years have gone by now, and the memories of diabetes grow fainter with each passing year. Only the small daily doses of maintenance immunosuppression medications I take to prevent my transplanted organs from failing, and vestiges of the neuropathy in my legs, mark me as someone who had diabetes. My vision is nearly perfect and with feeling back in my feet, I drive, bicycle, hike, canoe—activities many take for granted, but which I had lost to diabetes. My skin no longer has the fragile feel it had when I was diabetic. Cuts heal. And then there are the freedoms with food. When I look at restaurant menus, I no longer gravitate to items that "work." Now I choose what I *want* to eat. Food is a pleasure.

Last spring Tom and I were married on a boat as we cruised around Manhattan in its jeweled evening splendor. With a future of health before us, we had enough confidence to give freely to a friendship that we had both known could be a lasting and profound union. As we drifted under the same bridges I had seen from my bed in the cardiac intensive-care unit three years earlier, I realized how close I had come to never knowing that magical feeling of sharing my life with my husband. Tom travels extensively for work, and I often go with him. There is a new joy in going to Europe and Asia. Multiple time zones don't worry me. Tom and I laugh as I close my eyes and point at a line of Japanese writing on the menu and say, "I'll have one of those."

Diabetes, however, continues to be a shaping force in my life. Once my body was free of the disease I could look back, without protective rose-colored glasses, over my years as an insulin-dependent diabetic. Now I understand the progression of my disease, and I understand that from the day I was first diagnosed in 1970, I was on a path that would only get more difficult over time. During those years that I was healthy and active with insulin, glucose monitoring, and diet, I didn't stop to wonder who those people were who suffered diabetic blindness, amputation, heart attacks, and kidney failure. Now I know that they are—as I had been—the healthy diabetics of previous years.

Several years ago, I embarked on a professional relationship with diabetes and now work full time as the executive director of the Insulin-Free World Foundation, the nonprofit organization my husband and I founded at the end of 1996. Our work is devoted to providing comprehensive and current information via the Internet and printed newsletters. We act as an information exchange among diabetes clinicians, researchers, nurse educators, insurance professionals, government agencies, nonprofit organizations, and diabetic people. I hope to ease the burden for those who are on the path that I was on, to provide information about advances in science to make their lives as healthy as possible. Young diabetic people today can ground their ambitions and dreams in a reality that we did not have ten years ago—that there are alternatives to the disabling consequences of diabetes. And medicine is advancing rapidly; indeed, pancreas transplants and immunosuppression are safer today than they were when I had my surgery.

Much of the time I work to overcome insurance obstacles for people who want pancreas transplants and are already in the throes of secondary diabetic complications. Diabetic people have the right to know their options so that they can effectively manage their disease on both a day-to-day basis and over the long term. As diabetics, we depend on a broad range of medical professionals, but there is always more to know than can be learned in a doctor's office. I like to read. For years my bookshelf has been stacked with diabetes-maintenance manuals, reference books, and magazines, but in 1990 when I first heard that there were people who had found a way to be free of insulin-dependent diabetes, I could find little in my layperson's literature about my options. The few notations I did find made no distinction between the viability of pancreas transplants or the hunt for effective nasal insulin.

When I developed diabetic kidney disease, my doctors, books, and magazines were unanimous that my best bet would be to supplement my insulin- and glucose-monitoring regime with low-protein diets, blood-pressure medication, and dialysis. In fact, not one of the entourage of doctors who had taken care of me over the years ever told me there was an alternative. Even as I was poignantly aware that my health was deteriorating, and that insulin injections with frequent glucose monitoring were no longer able to stop the decline, I waited for that "Eureka" moment when *the* cure would free me.

When I learned, from my mother's chance encounter on her tireless hunt to rid me of diabetes, that a pancreas transplant might be a solution for me, I was excited, relieved, and frustrated all at once. I worked on Wall Street, and anyone I knew there who might have been diabetic was hiding it as well as I was, so I just muddled through. Only after I delved into the world of diabetes that lay hidden behind politics, the media, commercialism, and health-management organizations, did I realize fully that I had accepted a life of restrictions and ill health based on biased and misleading information. My blind and innocent ignorance was the catalyst to the Insulin-Free World Foundation's goal to provide information to help diabetic people, their families and friends to reach a better understanding of the disease that is rarely discussed.

Not long ago I attended an informal gathering that provided a particularly explicit image of diabetes today. The one hundred or so guests who assembled on that cold winter night were the most desperate of our kind—and they were looking for something, anything that might free them from their disease.

The guests stepped cautiously from the darkness outside into the brightly lit foyer of an elegant old townhouse on New York's Upper East Side. As I greeted them I couldn't help but think that we could have been any guests at any party—almost. With practiced nonchalance, I leaned against a chair to avoid losing my balance and staggering like a "drunken" sailor. I no longer wear leg braces, and I have the feeling back in my legs and feet that neuropathy had stolen, but still my balance is impaired. I noticed that one woman kept her balance by staying fused to her husband's arm. One gentleman sat over to the side with his bandaged foot in an orthopedic shoe. I watched him measuring his predicament against that of the young woman whose wheelchair was pushed into the high-ceilinged room. A young man, introduced to me when I came in as Kevin, "enjoyed" a glass of orange juice after what I imagined was a long day at work. I noticed that his hands were shaking almost imperceptibly. He was engaged in conversation with two of my supportive pretransplant friends, Jeff and Susan. Jeff, I knew, had a glass eye. Susan was blind, yet free of diabetes since her transplant.

In the room that evening were parents of diabetic children who already knew the desperation of living with the disease that, despite their meticulous efforts, was oftentimes unmanageable. Several had traveled to the city from the suburbs and even from neighboring states. With a voice that resonated with frustration, one of the fathers told me how he'd recently caught a glimpse of his teenage son angrily throwing an insulin syringe across his room. He'd walked on by, leaving his son's struggle buried there in that unreconciled moment, because he had no meaningful comfort to offer. I knew as he silently surveyed the room he was praying that his son would not end up like these people at the townhouse whose bodies had been ravaged by their vicious disease.

All too often during the years that I lived with diabetes I'd felt responsible for my deterioration. I was conditioned to believe that diabetes is manageable and that preventing its secondary complications was simply a matter of controlling blood-sugar levels. But as I looked around the room I wondered who outside the diabetic community ever sees these undercover lives. Who sees the children furtively hiding in school closets to inject insulin and to draw blood from their fingers? Or the young professionals secretly pushing insulin needles through their clothes under their desks? And when spouses wake up in the night to find their loved ones sweaty and corpselike in a coma at their side, where are those who believe that diabetes is a manageable disease? When diabetic complications set in, who remembers the simple joys of childhood that were abandoned to prevent them? Yet still we believe that we should do better. Self-conscious about our differences, we hide the tools of dialysis beneath long sleeves and baggy clothes. We hide our poor vision behind sarcastic or humorous excuses of "old age" or "too much sex," and we blame "uncomfortable shoes" for clumsy feet that have been broken and numbed by diabetic neuropathy. And we endure caustic glances and comments about "having a few too many" when we lose our balance, or when our eyes don't adjust from light to dark and we stumble or look confused. Dispersed among the blissfully unaware public, we can conceal the horrors that hide in the private moments of our lives; but concentrated in one place as we were on that wintry evening, the human toll was clear and the culprit was exposed.

Fran, a glowing example of the success of pancreas transplantation, was unable to make it to our gathering that evening because her father was dying of diabetes; she sat in a hospital room comforting him as he lay motionless in the bed. His feet were black. All day long his skin itched as he faded in and out of consciousness. Seven different specialists tried to help, but they had no more medicines or remedies in their arsenal. As her father moved toward death, Fran wrestled with the supreme paradox that after living with diabetes for more than twenty years, she was "cured." That night as we all talked excitedly about the almost unthinkable reality that there can be life after diabetes, Fran's father died. What a difference a generation of science had made.

This was very much on my mind that evening as I thought about what my generation of diabetics could lose by not knowing when to intervene in the life cycle of diabetes—by not knowing when the risks of continuing on insulin are greater than the risks of a transplant. We learn about day-to-day blood-sugar management and how to treat complications, but as diabetes progresses and the chaos of secondary complications is introduced, these familiar strategies are as helpful as rearranging furniture on the *Titanic*. We aren't given enough information to know about the course of diabetes, about new treatments and research, of policy and health-care reform, or of insurance, funding, and organ allocation. We don't know enough to steer clear of the iceberg.

I thought about my friends who had been lost to diabetes:

Victor, Bob, Debbie, and Michael. And as I heard my name being called by the evening's host to go to the podium to share my story, my thoughts flashed back to the meeting in London where I had made a presentation to the Asian brokerage companies. As I moved to the front of the room I thought about how far I had traveled from that blurry, shaky, sweaty time when the world went black immediately after my talk.

This time my thoughts were clear, my vision focused, and my sense of control intact; yet I was among fellow travelers, still searching. I, too, long for the day when cures for diabetes are safe enough to give back to diabetic children the spontaneity of their childhoods, and I hope for safer ways to prevent the rejection of transplanted organs. I yearn for a day when everyone who lives with this disease can say, "I *had* diabetes."

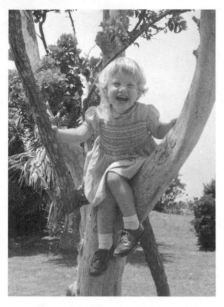

My idyllic childhood in Bermuda.

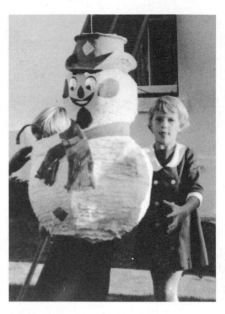

My snowman piñata.

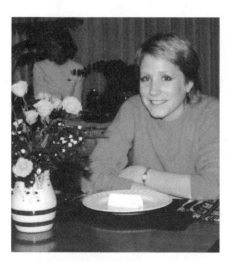

Another birthday cake that would end up in the garbage.

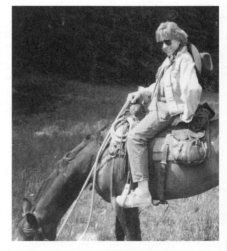

On the waiting list for my first kidney and pancreas transplant. It was difficult to ride because I couldn't feel my legs.

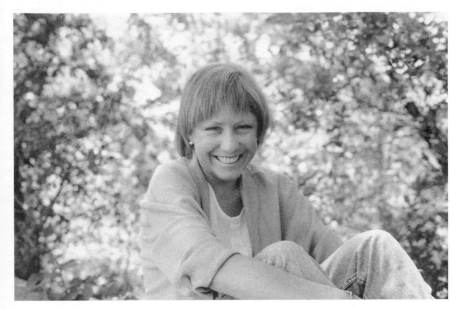

Two weeks after my pancreas-kidney transplant in Minneapolis.

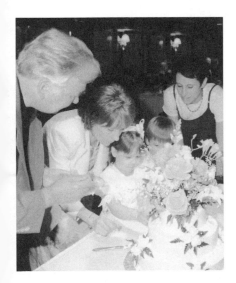

Having my cake and eating it, too.

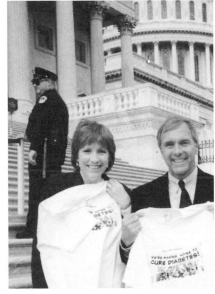

Me with Congressman George Nethercutt raising awareness of the need to cure diabetes.

Part II

An Insulin-Free World

Prologue

The experiences I have recounted in the first part of this book are personal anecdotes, threads in the story line of any diabetic person. Part 2 gives a wider perspective on diabetes to show how the frontiers of science—pancreas and islet transplantation, advances in immunology, cell engineering, and xenotransplantation—together with health-care policy, research funding, and social perception influence the health and choices of diabetic people.

My work has given me the opportunity to interact with a comprehensive spectrum of people from the industries and professions that serve the diabetic community—from advocates and government officials who strive to make sense of the complex needs of diabetics, to insurance professionals who calculate and quantify the economic cost of each physical insult that diabetes deals. Yet most valuable to me are my diabetic friends and colleagues who share their experiences with me and lead me to a better understanding of my own life with diabetes. It was a long road to discovering that diabetes, not I, was wrong, and that I was simply a casualty of diabetes' progression. I have met diabetic people in China, Australia, Germany, France, Canada, Puerto Rico, Thailand, Russia; indeed, in more than twenty different countries. Communication flows freely, perhaps because our differences are less important than our similarities—perhaps because we face a mutual enemy.

In the larger diabetic community, people are somewhat compartmentalized. Medical professionals attend seminars to share data with other medical professionals. Members of the insurance industry meet to develop coverage policies and analyze the trade-off between cost and quality of life. Nurse educators have their conferences to find ways to teach people who live with diabetes how to maximize the benefits of diabetes treatments. At the Insulin-Free World Foundation we make sure that knowledge developed in all these areas is available to diabetic people. Most important, we ensure that *our* experience of actually living with diabetes from day to day is integrated into the strategies and policies of the factions that influence our choices. Our two-pronged approach is to (1) get information to people and (2) urge people to use that information to raise public awareness for the urgent need to cure diabetes.

The following chapters on insulin therapy, pancreas transplantation, islet transplantation, and the role of society, politics, and economics are brief looks at issues at the forefront of that effort.

Chapter 11

Birth of a Chronic Disease

They [waves] are not located at a specific point. The crest of a
wave may move along with a given velocity, but the wave itself
is spread over the extended region between successive crests.
—*James Trefil,* Atoms to Quarks

L earning about diabetes has been analogous to peeling
back the layers of an onion, and now, as the twentieth
century draws to a close, an almost complete cross-
sectional anatomy is finally revealed. To put today's diabetes
treatments and research in context, it is worth taking the time
to ponder the first forays through the outer layers of the
onion.

The name *diabetes* comes from the Greek word meaning
"siphon" because its symptoms are excessive thirst and uri-
nation, as if the body were siphoning water. The disease was
recognized in the first century by a Greek physician who
described it as "the melting down of flesh and limbs into

urine." The first clue that diabetes had something to do with glucose wasn't found until 1674, when the English physician Dr. Thomas Willis tasted the urine of one of his severely diabetic patients and noticed that it was thick and sweet. A century later another English doctor, Matthew Dobson, used a simple hand-held kettle over an open fire to boil the urine of one of his diabetic patients. He found that when the water from the specimen evaporated, a sugary, crystalline residue remained. From then on he weighed the sugary extract from the urine of all of his diabetic patients to quantify the degree to which they were affected by the disease.[1] During that time, the surgeon general of the British artillery, Dr. John Rollo, was learning everything he could about diabetes to help a Captain Meredith, who was dying of the disease. He took diligent notes of what the captain ate, how much he weighed, and how often he urinated. Learning of Dobson's work, Dr. Rollo started taking routine measurements of the sugar in Captain Meredith's urine and realized that its quantity always increased after the captain ate starchy food. Although these discoveries were essential stepping stones to the treatments that would follow, they were of little practical benefit to people who were dying of diabetes.

Doctors felt the need to do something to help, but it was an era of ignorance in medicine. Because doctors did not know why diabetes caused sugar to be wasted in the urine of starving diabetics, their prescriptions and advice often caused more harm than good. Some physicians prescribed

[1]Rachmiel Levine, "The Endocrine Pancreas, Past and Present." In *Advances in Experimental Medicine and Biology,* vol. 124, ed. D. M. Klachko et al. (New York and London: Plenum Press, 1977), 1–13.

opium to relieve the pain. Others hoped that by eating bags of simple sugar diabetics could make up for what was lost in the urine, but this sad and hopeless act only hastened death.

To provide effective treatments, diabetologists and researchers needed to understand what in the beautifully complex human body had gone awry. In 1889, at the University of Strasbourg Medical Clinic, Oscar Minkowski, an assistant to Dr. Bernard Naunyn, the leading diabetes expert in Europe, and Joseph Von Mering, a pharmacologist by training, had the first major insight into the cause of diabetes. Minkowski and Von Mering were engaged in a debate about the role that pancreatic enzymes play in the digestion of fat, so they decided to remove the pancreas of a dog to study how the absence of pancreatic enzymes would affect digestion.

At that point, a serious illness in Von Mering's family required him to be away for a few days, so Minkowski was left to monitor the dog. The dog kept urinating on the floor and, as legend has it, the behavior attracted Minkowski's attention when a mass of flies congregated on the urine. Having worked as Dr. Naunyn's assistant, and being himself a good diabetologist, Minkowski suspected the dog was diabetic and confirmed his suspicions by testing the urine for sugar using a copper solution. Realizing that the dog had become diabetic when its pancreas was removed was the finding that finally linked diabetes to the pancreas.

It is interesting that Minkowski tried putting a small piece of pancreas beneath the dog's skin to see if he could cure the dog's diabetes; so even then, more than a century ago, Minkowski performed the first experiment with pancreas, indeed islet, transplantation. Years later Minkowski was quoted in a speech as saying, "A piece of scientific research may actually profit from the total ignorance on the part of the investigators. . . . Looking back convinces me that this ignorance was the real source of our success!"[2] But Minkowski was an expert on diabetes, and this was a classic example of a prepared mind taking advantage of serendipity.

Twenty years earlier, Paul Langerhans, a medical student in Berlin, had observed some previously unidentified cells scattered among the "exocrine" tissue in the pancreas of a rabbit. Without the insights of Minkowski and Von Mering that would follow, Langerhans was unable to explain the function of the cells he had discovered so he simply recorded his observation of the "little heaps of cells"[3] without assigning them a purpose. Before Langerhans' observation, the pancreas was believed to have only exocrine cells and so it was assumed that it had only an "exocrine" function, that is, the function of secreting external digestive juices. In 1893 Langerhans' clusters of cells piqued the curiosity of the French histologist Edouard Laguesse. Laguesse argued that the existence of the mysterious cells suggested that, in addition to the exocrine function, the pancreas might also produce a secretion that functioned within the organ. The "little heaps of cells," he suggested, might produce the internal secretion that performs the endocrine function. Laguesse named these cells the islets of Langerhans.

Often science develops in waves that build on prior dis-

[2]Oscar Minkowski, "Perspectives in Diabetes: Historical Development of the Theory of Pancreatic Diabetes," trans. and with introduction by Rachmiel Levine, *Diabetes* 38 (January 1989): 1–6.

[3]Rachmiel Levine, "The Endocrine Pancreas," 4.

coveries, with understanding coming more rapidly as knowledge accumulates and propels science forward. By the beginning of the twentieth century the synthesis of theories from the prior three centuries had started to form a meaningful profile of diabetes. Langerhans' observation of the islets, Minkowski's linking of the pancreas to diabetes, and Laguesse's hypothesis about the function of the islets led to the conclusion that the islets of Langerhans produce a secretion that must play a role in blood-sugar regulation.

By 1920 between 0.5 and 2 percent of the population of industrialized countries had diabetes.[4] Hospital wards were set up to isolate the sickly sweet smell of the wasting bodies of diabetics, and wards filled with young people whose fat, muscle, and vital organs were being consumed for energy by their digestive systems, a process known as ketoacidosis. Gasping and laboring to exhale the carbon dioxide that built up in their lungs, they slipped into comas and died. More diabetics were brought in, and the sickly sweet smell and gasping continued.

Hundreds of patients like these were brought to Dr. Frederick Allen at the Physiatric Institute in Morristown, New Jersey, and Dr. Elliot Joslin at his clinic in Boston, the two leading American diabetologists in the early part of the twentieth century. Dr. Allen concluded that the presence of sugar in the urine of diabetics was caused by an inability to convert the glucose derived from food into energy. In an effort to decrease the excess glucose, he prescribed a diet of four hundred to six hundred calories per day with one day of fasting

[4]Michael Bliss, *The Discovery of Insulin* (Chicago: University of Chicago Press, 1982), 21.

each week. Even though Dr. Allen's "starvation diet" was able to extend the lives of some of his diabetic patients for several years, diabetes was still a death sentence. The diet was publicly criticized for merely prolonging the agony of death while plunging its victims into greater misery with inhuman restrictions. Nevertheless, it was the only treatment at the turn of the century, and it did extend the lives of many diabetic people by several years.

The existence of a glucose-lowering hormone that might cure diabetes was still hypothetical in 1909 when Jean de Meyer named the internal secretion of the islets of Langerhans "insulin," from *insula,* the Latin word for island. Several researchers came very close to finding insulin in the decade prior to its actual discovery. One such scientist was Israel Kleiner, a young American working at the Rockefeller Institute. By injecting a mixture of glucose and "antidiabetic" derivatives of ground-up fresh pancreases into diabetic dogs, he was able to improve the animals' response to glucose. From 1915 to 1919 during World War I, Kleiner's work was halted because the country's human and economic resources were devoted to the war effort where deaths from diabetes paled in comparison to death at the hands of fellow humans. But while one war was waged on the battlefields, diabetes' war continued in the bodies of its victims. Another generation died before the country's resources could once again be applied to medical research.

Shortly after the war, Dr. Fred Banting had the intriguing idea that by tying off the pancreatic ducts of a dog, he could decompose the acinar tissue of the pancreas, leaving only the islets of Langerhans. He believed that he could isolate the islets and extract insulin that could then be used to lower the amount of sugar in the blood of diabetics. In October of 1920 Banting went to Professor J. J. MacLeod at the University of Toronto to ask for the use of a lab and a young scientist to assist him in pursuing his idea. With reluctance and a great deal of skepticism, MacLeod offered Banting a very small laboratory and the support of an assistant for a few weeks of the summer. Charles Best signed on as Banting's assistant. In the summer of 1921 Banting and Best began extracting a substance they called "isletin" from decomposed pancreases. By injecting isletin into diabetic dogs, they succeeded in lowering the dogs' blood-glucose levels. Their most compelling preliminary data were embodied in a severely diabetic dog, Marjorie, who was kept alive all summer with isletin injections. Today the survival of one dog for several months and a small series of successfully treated animals would not be considered sufficient data to begin human trials, but in the 1920s the risks and rewards of intervention were profoundly different. The risk of diabetes was death within a few years; the potential reward of isletin was a lifetime cure. Banting implored Professor MacLeod to sanction the start of human trials of isletin but it wasn't until winter blanketed Toronto that MacLeod agreed.

Leonard Thompson, the fourteen-year-old boy who was the first person to undergo the experimental treatment, was admitted to the Toronto General Hospital as a charity ward case.[5] After following Allen Therapy for two years, Leonard

[5] F. G. Banting, C. H. Best, J. B. Collip, W. R. Campbell, and A. A. Fletcher, "Pancreatic Extracts in the Treatment of Diabetes Mellitus: Preliminary Report," *Canadian Medical Association Journal* 2 (March 1922): 141–146

had wasted away to a mere sixty-five pounds, his diet was a scant four hundred and fifty calories, and death was imminent. On January 11, 1922, Leonard Thompson became the first person to receive insulin. His arm turned red and swollen at the injection site, and the doctors noted with dismay that there was only a modest decline in Leonard's glucose level. James Collip, a biochemist who worked with Banting and Best, labored for five more days to find the precise concentration of alcohol in which to suspend the active ingredients in insulin while allowing the contaminating proteins in the crushed pancreas to settle out. For another week Collip tested the extract for potency and adverse local reactions. On January 23, when Collip was satisfied he had an effective, nontoxic solution, Leonard received his second dose.

Leonard's glucose levels dropped quickly, and his life-threatening ketoacidosis disappeared altogether. He became more animated and, with each sign of improvement, Leonard's father and doctors realized that this was an unprecedented advance—diabetes had been reduced from a fatal to a chronic disease. The press reported this sensational news accurately but doctors who hadn't personally witnessed the dramatic recoveries of diabetics treated with insulin were, at first, skeptical. Cautious physicians and "humanitarians" of all types warned that insulin caused diabetics to go into violent convulsions when too much was taken, that animals had been needlessly sacrificed, and that not a single person had been cured. Indeed, by our definition today, insulin did not cure diabetes. But for Leonard Thompson and millions of other diabetics, insulin made it possible to survive.

Chapter 12

Insulin Therapy

We've made some discoveries that would suggest there was an epistemologic collapse. . . . This was a classic example of how you can get caught up in a snowstorm of details learning more and more about less and less and let the great truth escape.

—*Dr. Thomas Starzl, professor of surgery,*
University of Pittsburgh[1]

The impetus behind the discovery of insulin was the need to lower blood-sugar levels to prevent death from diabetes. Beginning with the first insulin injection given to Leonard Thompson in 1922, the guiding principle of diabetes management has been to use insulin to control blood-sugar levels in people whose insulin-producing cells have been completely destroyed, or who have too few to maintain normal glucose metabolism. Natural insulin-producing cells, the beta cells in the islets of the pancreas, house

[1]B. D. Colen, "Organ Concert," *Time* 148, no. 4 (special issue, Fall 1996): 170.

a very complex system of responses that react spontaneously and precisely to each fluctuation of blood-sugar level—fluctuations that are provoked by all processes of living—physical, emotional, and psychological.

For more than a decade following its introduction, insulin was innocently heralded as a cure for diabetes, and indeed it had solved the most immediate problem of rapid death from the disease. It wasn't until those who had been spared by insulin had lived long enough to develop secondary complications that it became apparent that diabetes had not been cured.

With insulin as the only treatment for insulin-dependent diabetes for most of this century, the challenges of using it to control blood-sugar levels have, by necessity, dominated the teachings and activities of medical schools, nonprofit associations, pharmaceutical companies, and diabetes-specific government agencies. A number of studies have shown that strict blood-sugar control can delay the onset and slow the progression of secondary diabetic complications, but exogenous insulin cannot duplicate the refined mechanism of beta cells. Insulin was indeed a remarkable advance and has extended the lives of people with insulin-dependent diabetes twentyfold, but as we exit the twentieth century its shortcomings are sadly clear:

- Secondary complications of the eyes, nerves, and kidneys affect more than half of those people who survive more than twenty years with diabetes.[2]

[2]D. E. R. Sutherland, P. F. Gores, A. C. Farney et al., "Evolution of Kidney, Pancreas, and Islet Transplantation for Patients with Diabetes at the University of Minnesota," *American Journal of Surgery* 166 (1993): 456–91.

- Eighty percent of all persons who have had diabetes for fifteen years or more have evidence of damage to the small blood vessels in their eyes.[3]
- The risk of a leg amputation is fifteen to forty times greater for people who have diabetes. Each year more than 56,000 feet or legs are lost to diabetes.[4]
- Middle-aged people with diabetes have a death rate twice as high as their nondiabetic peers.[5]
- Cardiovascular disease is two to four times more common in people with diabetes.[6]
- Diabetes accounts for 40 percent of all new cases of end-stage renal disease.[7]
- One American is killed by diabetes every three minutes.[8]

In absolute numbers, there are as many as 120,000 new cases of blindness, kidney failure, or amputation per year resulting from diabetes. Every year diabetes contributes to 190,000 deaths.[9] What does that mean for a ten-year-old child who is diagnosed with diabetes today? In the first few years, that child's risk of suffering a complication or death is remote. Statistically, however, it is true that an additional 6

[3] American Academy of Ophthalmology, 1995, educational brochure.

[4] American Diabetes Association, *Diabetes Facts and Figures*, 1997.

[5] Centers for Disease Control and Prevention, *National Diabetes Fact Sheet: National Estimates and General Information on Diabetes in the United States* (Atlanta: U.S. Department of Health and Human Services, 1997).

[6] *National Diabetes Fact Sheet.*

[7] *National Diabetes Fact Sheet.*

[8] Juvenile Diabetes Foundation International, *Diabetes Facts* (1998).

[9] *National Diabetes Fact Sheet.*

million cases of serious complications or death will be reported in the diabetic population before that child turns thirty. With the passage of time, his or her risk of being among them shifts from unlikely to likely.

To chart the best course with diabetes, it helps to conceptualize how the disease can play out over the long term within the context of evolving medical treatments. Figure I illustrates this concept by using my characterization of the stages of diabetes. I think of the first stage as *nondiabetic*, that is, when a propensity exists but the metabolism has not yet been affected. I refer to those years after diagnosis, when a person does well with insulin injections, glucose monitoring, and diet, with no symptoms of complications, as a *condition*. When diabetes progresses to the early stages of eye, nerve, kidney, or heart disease, or hypoglycemic unawareness, I have labeled diabetes a *disease*. If blindness, amputation, or dialysis should occur, diabetes is in a stage that I call *disability*.

Figure I: Theoretical stages of diabetes and impact of advances in medical treatments

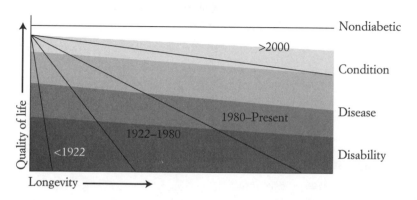

Improvements in the quality of life are represented on the vertical axis and longevity on the horizontal axis. Advances in medicine that increase either the longevity or quality of life shift the diabetic lifeline closer to that of the nondiabetic population. In 1922 the discovery of insulin caused a dramatic shift in the curve, increasing diabetics' life expectancy twentyfold. In the 1980s the introduction of blood-glucose monitors and the ability to practice better blood-sugar control delayed the onset and slowed the progression of secondary complications for some people. Similarly, laser technology and other microscopic eye procedures have reduced the incidence of severe vision loss and delayed the onset of eye complications.

Thinking beyond the day-to-day management of diabetes, the long-term goal for the individual must be to reach for advances in medicine that can increase longevity or improve the quality of life. From the time of diagnosis, diabetics chart a course to optimize both the quality of their days and the length of their lives. To determine if there will be an improvement in quality of life and/or longevity, people with diabetes need information about the benefits and risks of each new therapy to compare them to the benefits and risks of existing treatments. From 1983 to 1993, in an effort to compare the effects of "intensive" insulin therapy against those of "conventional" insulin therapy, the National Institutes of Health conducted a $280 million study called the Diabetes Control and Complications Trial (DCCT). The sheer number of people who survive with insulin-dependent diabetes is a testament to the incredible value of insulin, yet the DCCT went beyond that to show the possibilities and limitations of insulin therapy.

As defined for the study, "intensive" therapy consisted of three or more daily insulin injections or insulin pump therapy, four or more daily blood-glucose tests, frequent dietary instruction, monthly clinic visits with a diabetes treatment team (physician, nurse educator, dietitian, and behavioral therapist), and weekly telephone calls. "Conventional" therapy consisted of one or two insulin injections daily, visits with the diabetes treatment team every three months, and daily urine tests or blood-glucose monitoring.

The project began in 1983 with 278 participants. The first two years were devoted to planning and feasibility studies. Because intensive therapy caused a high incidence of severe hypoglycemia (dangerously low blood-sugar levels) during the feasibility studies, changes were made in the eligibility criteria to exclude from the full-scale trial anyone who had a history of severe hypoglycemia. The full cohort of 1,441 participants was achieved in 1989, four years before the study ended. The average follow-up was six and a half years.

In spite of excluding from the study people with a history of severe hypoglycemia, the incidence of severe hypoglycemia in the intensive therapy group was three times that of the conventional therapy group.[10] If you were to plot average blood sugars on a graph relative to the incidence of complications, the graph would show that long-term diabetic complications decrease, but don't stop, as average blood sugars improve. As average blood sugars approach normal levels

[10]Diabetes Control and Complications Trial Research Group, "The Effect of Intensive Treatment of Diabetes on the Development and Progression of Long-Term Complications in Insulin-Dependent Diabetes Mellitus," *New England Journal of Medicine* 329, no. 14 (1993): 977–86.

where long-term complications could be prevented, the risk of severe hypoglycemia increases significantly. This leaves only a brief window of opportunity where there is neither a risk of severe hypoglycemia or long-term progression to secondary diabetic complications.

Intensive insulin therapy was able to delay the onset and slow the progression of retinopathy, neuropathy, and nephropathy by 29 to 74 percent, but could not stop them from occurring. Complications did progress in the group of intensively managed patients, just not so quickly as in the conventionally managed group.[11] An analysis of the results of the trial published by the DCCT Research Group in 1996 reports that intensive therapy adds 7.7 additional years of sight, 5.8 additional years of kidney function, 5.6 additional years free from lower extremity amputation, and 5.1 years of life over conventional therapy.[12] Young children diagnosed with diabetes would therefore confront these problems in their thirties and forties instead of in their twenties or thirties.

The DCCT Research Group also reported that intensive therapy is not recommended for children under the age of thirteen, people with heart disease or advanced complications, the elderly, and people with a history of frequent or severe hypoglycemia. As Dr. David Nathan, a senior member of the DCCT Research Group wrote to me, "We tried to

[11]The DCCT Research Group, "The Effect of Intensive Treatment of Diabetes."

[12]Diabetes Control and Complications Trial Research Group, "Lifetime Benefits and Costs of Intensive Therapy as Practiced in the Diabetes Control and Complications Trial," *Journal of the American Medical Association* 276, no. 17 (1996): 1410–11.

determine the fraction of the Type 1 population in the U.S. that would fulfill the DCCT criteria on the basis of age, duration of diabetes, and other criteria. Approximately 17 percent of the entire Type 1 population appeared to fulfill those criteria." A treatment that benefits 17 percent of the Type 1 diabetic population is important, but obviously we need to find solutions beyond intensive diabetes management.

The DCCT was a six-and-a-half-year study of a select group of approximately 700 people (half of those enrolled) who practiced intensive therapy for a small period in their lifetime with diabetes. However, diabetes is a life-long disease that affects millions of people, and although the DCCT is generally regarded as one of the most flawlessly implemented clinical trials in the history of medicine, widespread success with the protocols used has yet to be realized in practice. The Diabetes Association (ADA) describes the DCCT as "the longest and largest study to show that lowering blood-glucose concentration to more normal levels through intensive treatment slows or prevents the development of diabetic complications."[13] I would argue that the longest, largest—and most persuasive—study of insulin therapy overall is the one that is conducted every day, every year, in the real lives of people with diabetes. The results of *this* study can be found in the cumulative national statistics that show ever-increasing incidences of blindness, amputation, heart attacks, and kidney disease.

The results achieved by the DCCT's intensive insulin-

[13]American Diabetes Association, Response to the DCCT. American Diabetes Association Web site, www.diabetes.org/adatx/adaresearch/dcct.asp/

therapy group have been disappointing in practice for a number of reasons: the increased risk of severe hypoglycemia; the burden of sustaining a regimen of multiple daily insulin injections, blood-glucose tests, and dietary restrictions; and the fact that intensive insulin therapy itself does not guarantee a life free of diabetic complications. As Dr. Alan Jacobson of the Joslin Diabetes Center and Harvard Medical School wrote in the *New England Journal of Medicine*, "Optimal treatment of IDDM [insulin-dependent diabetes mellitus] is difficult if not impossible in the case of most patients. For example, even in the DCCT, with a highly selected and motivated research population given ample resources and education, only five percent of patients maintained an average concentration of glycosylated hemoglobin in the target or normal range."[14] Indeed, the complete long-term subservience to bodily function that is required to manage diabetes goes beyond what can reasonably be defined as a "manageable" solution. Nevertheless, diabetics continue to be held accountable for the failures of an inadequate therapy:

WASHINGTON, June 23, 1998 (Associated Press)— The National Institutes of Health wants diabetics to remember that controlling blood sugar can sharply reduce complications from the disease. "People with diabetes need to step forward and take control of their diabetes," Dr. Philip Gordon, director of NIH's National Institute of Diabetes and Digestive and Kidney Diseases, said in a statement . . . .

[14]Alan Jacobson, "The Psychological Care of Patients with Insulin-Dependent Diabetes Mellitus," *New England Journal of Medicine* 334, no. 19 (1996): 1249–53.

Dr. Gordon's remarks were made as part of an ongoing multimedia campaign of public-service announcements on radio and television, in print, and through various "partnership" organizations and educational materials. It was the first such public program initiated by the National Diabetes Education Program (NDEP), created in June of 1997 by the National Institute of Diabetes and Digestive and Kidney Diseases (NIDDK), itself an arm of the National Institutes of Health (NIH). The campaign, the result of one and a half years' worth of meetings between the NDEP and various public and private groups, sounded its theme with its public launch in the summer of 1998: "Through the NDEP," Dr. Gordon said, "we hope to get the message out that diabetes is serious, common, costly, and controllable."[15] And with perfect consistency, Dr. Frank Vinicor, director of the Division of Diabetes at the Center for Disease Control—another partner in the campaign—said at the June 23 press conference: "People with diabetes need to step forward and take control of their diabetes. Scientific studies provide compelling evidence that maintaining blood-sugar levels at less than 7 percent . . . may reduce the risk of diabetes complications by 50 to 80 percent." [16]

People who live with insulin-dependent diabetes know that good blood-sugar control is better than poor blood-sugar control, but although insulin, glucose tests, diet, and exercise are *necessary* to manage diabetes, they are by no means *sufficient*. Some people need only moderately good blood-sugar control to prevent complications; others need

[15]NIDDK and CDC, press release, June 22, 1998.
[16]NIDDK and CDC, press release, June 23, 1998.

perfect control, but as the DCCT showed, perfect control is rarely achieved—even with intensive insulin therapy. As Dr. David Sutherland, the director of the Diabetes Institute at the University of Minnesota, says, "Metabolic control *and* genetic susceptibility to individual complications play a role; if genetic susceptibility is high, the degree of metabolic control needed to prevent secondary complications may be impossible or unacceptably burdensome."[17]

Sue Schaible, one of the editorial staff for *Insulin-Free-TIMES*, the quarterly newsletter of the Insulin-Free World Foundation, sent me the following letter by e-mail. Both Sue and her son Derek have diabetes, and her letter illustrates my point. "I am so upset," she began.

Derek's sugars have been running between 100 and 200 with no lows for the past week and a half. I was quite pleased. Before he went to bed last night, about two hours after his snack, his sugar was 170. This past week it was usually a little lower than that, about 140 to 150, but I decided that was okay. I had an uneasy feeling around 12:30 A.M. so I checked his sugar. It was 98. I woke him up feeling that he'd gone down too fast and too far. I wondered about the swimming that he did earlier in the afternoon, even though it was only for an hour and he had the usual snack beforehand without any problems later. He said he wanted some frozen yogurt, which I gave him. A short while later he was also drinking juice which I thought was a bit much, but I didn't say anything because

[17]David E. R. Sutherland, "Today's Solutions for Type 1 Diabetes: Pancreas Transplantation," paper given at Insulin-Free World Foundation seminar, St. Louis, Mo., May 16, 1998.

I've often said something to him about extra food and then found him ending up going low. So I let him finish the juice as well, brush his teeth again, and back to bed. Around 3 A.M. he was sleeping and seemed fine. At 6:30 A.M. I walked into his room asking how he was as I usually do. Instead of his normal response of "Good morning," he screamed and I noticed he was having seizures. I immediately grabbed the Glucagon and injected him with it and the seizures resolved in only a few minutes. But those few minutes felt like a lifetime of grief while I wondered if he would come back completely. All from "good" control. This is so wrong. This is unacceptable. I can't bear to lose my child who gives so much. This is a child whose primary concerns in life are convincing me to let him have a lizard for a pet (which he hasn't done, yet), and playing the piano well enough for the people at the nursing home to enjoy his visits!

My heart sank to hear Derek say "I know I should be exercising more, I was told I should be exercising more because it would help my diabetes." Even though he is a child in the midst of the freedom of summer, his play has become exercise that must be planned, preceded by food and monitored with blood tests. I'm so thankful he is alive—but for his undeserved suffering now, and yet to be, today will be a day of tears for me.

The American Diabetes Association is articulating a widespread philosophy in reporting that "Individuals affected by diabetes must learn self-management skills and make lifestyle changes to effectively manage diabetes and avoid or delay the complications associated with this disorder. For these reasons, self-management education is the cornerstone of treatment for all people with diabetes."[18] Certainly, control is important. Yet the philosophy that life-style changes and management skills are sufficient to control blood-sugar levels establishes a standard that condemns many with uncontrollable diabetes to failure. Likewise, the expectations that have been propagated by the DCCT obscure the truth that diabetes is the problem, not the people who have it.

Treatments for diabetes have made only modest advances since insulin's dramatic entrance in the 1920s. Intensive insulin therapy, new delivery systems, better glucose monitors and treatments for secondary complications help improve daily life but hold little promise of a significant shift in either quality or longevity of life over the long term. Today, more than five years after the DCCT was published in the *New England Journal of Medicine*, 10 to 15 percent of the insulin-dependent diabetic population—just shy of the 17 percent who are eligible—is practicing intensive insulin therapy.[19] Still, there is no solution for the majority of people who live with diabetes. Nor is there any improvement in the overall impact of diabetes on society. Clinical and research advances in immunology and transplantation in the last decade have put cures for diabetes within reach. It is time to make *curing* diabetes our top research priority.

[18]American Diabetes Association, "Clinical Practice Recommendations 1998, National Standards for Diabetes Self-Management Education Program and American Diabetes Association Review Criteria," *Diabetes Care* 21 (suppl. 1).

[19]Z.T. Bloomgarden, "American Diabetes Association Postgraduate Course, 1996: Treatment and Prevention of Diabetes," *Diabetes Care* (1996): 784.

Chapter 13

Pancreas Transplantation

This "telephone" has too many shortcomings to be seriously considered as a means of communication. The device is inherently of no value to us.

—*Western Union internal memo, 1876*

"Do you think a pancreas transplant is a cure for diabetes?" I asked Dr. Sutherland, the transplant surgeon who performed my kidney-pancreas transplant. "Well, if you equate 'cure' with insulin independence, you could use the term for pancreas transplants," he explained, "but I would not. I look on pancreas transplants today as a better treatment, or at least a treatment that induces insulin independence. A cure for me would be insulin independence without the need for ongoing treatment with drugs."

Yet I refer to my pancreas transplant as *my* cure. Sure, it isn't a cure for everyone, but it was, as the dictionary would say, a "means of healing, restoring [me] to health, a remedy." To that extent I am cured. My secondary complications have reversed, I have a normally functioning pancreas, and normal glucose metabolism. "Do you think 'cure' is subjective?" I asked, "or do you think it has an absolute definition?"

"Deb, I look on it as a matter of precision and not subjectivity. You are cured of insulin dependence, but not diabetes per se. The latter is just treated. To me you have a choice of treatments—immunosuppression drugs or exogenous insulin. If you stop the drugs, you will have to take insulin; if you take insulin, you don't need the drugs. If you didn't need either, you'd be cured of diabetes"—he paused—"or perhaps at least if you didn't need to do anything actively to sustain that state. A pancreas transplant only cures insulin dependence and some secondary complications; it *is* a superior treatment though in terms of diabetic control and ease of management."

"So, if being insulin independent and immunosuppression free required surgery and a single dose of immunosuppression that lasted a lifetime, it would satisfy your definition of a cure because no ongoing treatment would be required, right?"

"Yes. That's right," he said.

"I think of a pancreas transplant with immunosuppression as the first solution in the era of *cures* for diabetes because an evolution of this approach could lead to a maintenance-free state—a universal cure," I suggested. "I think of superior *treatments* as evolutions in conscious diabetes management—when a person has to think how much insulin to administer or food to eat. Perhaps cures for me are solutions that put an end to the metabolic defect."

"Deb, think of it like a broken bone. When it heals, you are cured of the fracture, but if you need a brace, you still have bone disease—you are just cured of crutches. I think a diabetes cure is possible with a pancreas transplant, or with beta cell regeneration. It is just not there yet without an ongoing need for immunosuppression drugs."

"But even without the need for ongoing drugs, it is always possible that the transplanted pancreas could be lost to thrombosis [blood clotting] or infection. Then the cure would be only temporary—like a remission."

"It is a fine point. If it thrombosed, it would cause a recurrence of diabetes; the cure would have been temporary. I think a pancreas transplant without immunosuppression, which may soon be possible, is a cure."

"I hope so," I said, "because even though I think of my pancreas transplant as *my* cure for diabetes, I look forward to a day when I don't need to take immunosuppression drugs."

"The reason I am careful with the word *cure* is that it can inflate people's hopes beyond what can be done now. For a lot of people, a cure has more requirements than what we can achieve at this time. Deb, this is mainly semantics, but it is important for people to think about these things when they look at their options with transplantation."

"I don't know which box to check on medical questionnaires when they ask, 'Diabetes: yes or no?' Usually I make an extra box for 'history of diabetes.' The other day when I went to see my doctor in New York, the nurse checked my blood sugar out of habit. It was my normal 81 milligrams per deciliter, but because she'd forgotten I'm not diabetic anymore, she gave me some cookies to stop my blood sugar going too low! I didn't say anything because the cookies were delicious," I smiled.

"It is hard to find good cookies," Dr. Sutherland said with his dry sense of humor.

For thousands of us who have suffered from the secondary complications of diabetes, pancreas transplantation has given us back years of health. Indeed, it is currently the only consistently successful means for insulin-dependent diabetics to achieve normal blood-sugar levels; yet being a pancreas recipient requires medical management too. Individuals need to know what the trade-offs are between continuing with diabetes and getting a new pancreas.

The pancreas is a long, narrow organ weighing approximately 3 ounces (90 grams) and is located below the liver and behind the stomach. It is attached to the main blood vessel running through the abdomen and to the first portion of the intestine after the stomach, the duodenum. Ninety-eight percent of the pancreas consists of exocrine tissue, which secretes digestive enzymes. The remaining 1 to 2 percent is accounted for by the clusters of cells that make up the islets of Langerhans (islets). These clusters consist predominantly of insulin-producing beta cells. A person becomes diabetic when these cells are destroyed by his or her immune system. The goal of pancreas transplantation is to replace these insulin-producing beta cells. To date, replacing them as part of a segmental (piece of) or whole pancreas organ has been the only consistent means to normalize blood-sugar levels without any further need for exogenous insulin.

There are a number of ways to approach pancreas transplantation: simultaneously with a kidney transplant (SPK), after a kidney transplant (PAK), or as a pancreas transplant alone (PTA). Most pancreas transplants are done in conjunction with kidney transplants because patients with end-stage kidney disease must already undergo surgery and take immunosuppression drugs. More than 85 percent of the pancreas transplants done today are SPKs, approximately 10 percent are PAKs, and the remainder are PTAs.[1] In any of these procedures, the kidney and pancreas are transplanted into the abdominal cavity; the native organs, the person's birth organs, are left in place.

For a subset of the diabetic population, receiving a successful pancreas transplant has caused a substantial leap to a higher quality of life and greater longevity. Since doctors William Kelly and Richard Lillehei performed the first pancreas transplant at the University of Minnesota in 1966, approximately eleven thousand transplants have been reported worldwide. Since 1994 more than one thousand such operations have been performed every year with overall success rates (insulin independence at one year after transplant) from 1994–1997 at 83 percent, equivalent to the success rate of kidney transplants alone in diabetic patients.[2] Still, the option of pancreas transplantation is relatively unknown to the diabetic population with its greatest proponents being those who have witnessed its success firsthand.

It was Sir Peter Medawar and his collaborators in the 1940s and 1950s who demonstrated in mice and chickens that rejection of "non-self" donor tissue can be prevented if

---

[1] *International Pancreas Transplant Registry* 10, no. 1 (May 1998).
[2] *International Pancreas Transplant Registry* 10, no. 1 (May 1998).

cells from that non-self tissue are introduced into the recipient during neonatal life.[3] This work established the immunological basis for transplantation and won Medawar the Nobel Prize in medicine in 1960. On July 3, 1950, *Time* magazine carried a report of the first human organ transplant: "Last week in Chicago, trying a desperate experiment on a woman doomed to die because both kidneys were hopelessly diseased, doctors performed the first human kidney transplanting on record." The story was about Ruth Tucker and the bold, last-ditch attempt of doctors R. H. Lawler and J. W. West to save her life. Eight months after her transplant, Mrs. Tucker's urine output slowed and exploratory surgery showed a dark cavity where the transplanted kidney should have been. On June 11, 1951, *Time* magazine carried a follow-up article reporting that the operation had failed. It quoted Dr. P. H. McNulty, one of the surgeons on the team, as saying, "The grafted kidney was not functioning and never had. It had shrunk to the size of a hazelnut. The reason," Dr. McNulty explained, "was that the donor's tissues were incompatible with Mrs. Tucker's."

On December 23, 1954, Dr. Joseph Murray (who would receive the Nobel Prize in medicine in 1990) performed the first successful human organ transplant in the history of medicine at Peter Bent Brigham Hospital in Boston. The recipient was a young man named Richard Herrick, who was suffering from kidney failure. Richard had been blessed with

[3]L. Brent, R. Billingham, A. Mitchison, L. Thomas, and D. Pyke, "Sir Peter B. Medawar: An Outstanding Contribution to Medical Science," in *History of Transplantation: Thirty-Five Recollections*, ed. P. Terasaki (Los Angeles: UCLA Tissue Typing Laboratory, 1991), 3–5.

an identical twin brother and, even though there had been no successes with human organ transplantation, his doctors believed that Richard's twin brother could donate a kidney that Richard's immune system would accept as "self." The kidney worked perfectly for nine years before it failed—not from rejection, but from the recurrence of his original disease. As Dr. Murray wrote in his recollections, "It was spying into the future because we had achieved our long-term goal by bypassing, but not solving, the issue of biological incompatibility." Nevertheless, Richard's prolonged life marked a milestone in the history of medicine.

It was a time of many firsts in transplantation. In 1966, the same year that the first pancreas transplant was performed in Minnesota, so too was the first intestinal transplant. A year later, the South African surgeon Dr. Christiaan Barnard performed the first heart transplant in Cape Town. The patient, Louis Washkansky, lived for eighteen days. That same year, Dr. Thomas Starzl performed the first successful liver transplant in Denver for Julie Rodriguez, a nineteen-month-old child who lived for four hundred extra days. And in 1968, Dr. F. Derom of Louvain Medical Center in Brussels performed the first successful lung transplant.

In the mid-1960s dialysis and kidney transplantation emerged as treatments for kidney failure, but not for people with diabetes. Diabetic people with kidney disease were rarely accepted for dialysis because the survival rate was dismal for those who had tried it—but their chances of surviving without it were zero. They were also excluded from kidney transplant programs because many doctors believed that the lifelong regimen of steroids required to prevent transplanted kidneys from rejecting would send blood sugars spiraling out of control. Because doctors generally believed that diabetic people had a natural propensity to infection, it was feared that immunosuppression would increase that susceptibility. Yet without attempting a transplant, diabetics had no chance of survival. Later in the 1960s researchers discovered that diabetic people are not predisposed to infection, but that infections are a function of blood-sugar levels. Furthermore, if insulin is adjusted to the steroid-induced increase in production of blood sugar by the liver, steroids could be administered without worsening blood-sugar control. In the absence of that knowledge, though, the limited and expensive resources for dialysis and transplant programs were allocated to nondiabetic patients whose survival rates were thought to be better than those of diabetic patients. Diabetic patients with kidney failure were mostly left to die.[4]

During that time when there seemed to be no hope for people with diabetic kidney disease, doctors Lillehei and Kelly reasoned that by transplanting a pancreas in addition to a kidney they could eliminate diabetes altogether. Steroids could then be administered just as for nondiabetic patients. The first pancreas transplant worked for a brief time. For the first time in the long history of diabetes, a person with insulin-dependent diabetes was able to achieve normal glucose metabolism without the use of insulin. However, after three months, the recipient died of sepsis. Of the first fourteen pancreas transplants performed, only one functioned for

[4]D. E. R. Sutherland, P. F. Gores, A. C. Farney et al., "Evolution of Kidney, Pancreas, and Islet Transplantation for Patients with Diabetes at the University of Minnesota," *American Journal of Surgery* 166 (1993): 456–91.

more than a year without being rejected. Although most of the patients had become insulin independent right away, thirteen failed for technical reasons (primarily thrombosis and infection) or rejected the transplant within a few months.[5] The team at the University of Minnesota temporarily ceased doing pancreas transplants while they went back to the laboratory to improve surgical techniques and strategies to prevent rejection.

In the 1970s, the worldwide results of pancreas transplants were disappointing. By the close of the decade 102 pancreas transplants for 96 patients had been attempted, but the mortality rate was high, and fewer than 6 percent of the transplanted pancreases functioned for more than one year. The tide changed in the late 1970s when improved surgical techniques developed in the labs were ready for human trials. In 1978 pancreas transplants were resumed at the University of Minnesota. Dr. David Sutherland, a young Minnesota-born transplant surgeon who had followed doctors Lillihei and Kelly's work while he was in medical school, embarked on the first series of pancreas transplants to result in consistent success with the procedure. Dr. Sutherland stayed at the University of Minnesota and now heads the oldest and largest pancreas transplant program in the world.

During the 1980s pancreas transplantation evolved in labs and operating rooms in response to the immediate needs of their patients. Improvements came so quickly that those not intimately involved would have found it difficult to stay abreast of the advances, primarily from new ways to drain

[5]Sutherland et al., "Evolution of Kidney, Pancreas, and Islet Transplantation," p. 471.

the pancreas and more refined immunosuppression protocols.

The rising success rates for transplantation have been closely related to advances in immunology. In the early 1950s, steroids and radiation, the only known means to thwart the immune response, often led to fatal infections and toxicity. Logically the high risk of death resulted in transplantation being a last-ditch life-saving measure. The introduction of Imuran in the 1960s and Cyclosporine in the early 1980s increased the overall success rates of transplants and mitigated the side effects of immunosuppression. In 1994 and 1995, two new drugs, FK506 (also known as Tacrolimus or Prograf) and mycophenolate mofetil (CellCept), were introduced. Steroid doses have been greatly reduced and in many cases discontinued altogether. These drugs have not been used for long enough to make definitive statements about their long-term effects, but having a range of drugs to choose from has allowed for significantly more effective immunosuppression protocols using smaller, less toxic doses that cause less toxicity.

Dr. Thomas Starzl, the pioneer of liver transplantation, calls immunosuppression the "heart and soul and philosophy" of transplantation. Indeed, the introduction of FK506 and CellCept reduced the rejection of pancreases transplanted simultaneously with kidneys to just 2 percent, pancreases transplanted after kidneys to 9 percent, and pancreas transplants alone to 16 percent.[6] Technical failure has also dropped from 16 percent in the late 1980s to only 9 percent today. The success of pancreas transplantation has advanced at an astonishing rate, from fewer than 10 percent of the pan-

[6]*International Pancreas Transplant Registry* 10, no. 1 (May, 1998).

creas recipients achieving normal blood-sugar levels in the late 1970s to 70 percent in the mid-1980s. Data collected between 1994 and 1996 from pancreas transplants performed simultaneously with kidney transplants at U.S. hospitals show success rates of 86 percent. Yet because many of today's doctors are not aware that pancreas transplantation has developed into a routine therapy, they are reluctant to discuss it with their patients; many doctors still believe that the procedure is experimental. Often today's success rates are lost in statistics that average the early failures with current results; likewise, much of the commentary about complications associated with immunosuppression describes problems of a bygone era.

Dr. Paul Robertson, a professor in the Division of Metabolism, Endocrinology and Nutrition at the University of Washington and one of today's preeminent diabetologists, has studied hundreds of pancreas recipients. He says, "A transplanted pancreas brings a person closer to normal blood glucose control than any other method, better even than intensive insulin therapy. Transplanting a pancreas is no longer an experimental operation. It's the application of this procedure that remains controversial."[7] The application of pancreas transplantation alone, without a kidney, remains the most controversial. Unlike a pancreas transplant received in conjunction with a kidney where the benefits are freedom from both dialysis and diabetes management, the benefit of a pancreas transplant alone is freedom only from diabetes management. The controversy arises because many believe that insulin therapy is sufficient to manage diabetes.

The aggressive and revolutionary advances in immunology

[7]Marilyn Citron, "Why Wait?" *Diabetes Forecast* 49, no. 2 (1996).

and transplantation for treating diabetes seem to have caught the world by surprise. Many people try to slow the progression of secondary complications with the same, or similar, insulin regimens they were using when their complications developed. Relatively few know that pancreas transplantation is a successful therapy for kidney disease, hypoglycemic unawareness, and diabetes that cannot be controlled with insulin injections. People with insulin-dependent diabetes who today are being disabled by this disease are victims of "lag time," the time it takes for a new technology or treatment to be recognized and accepted as standard treatment by doctors and insurance carriers.

This period of lag time is reminiscent of the time immediately following the discovery of insulin. Then, physicians who had not witnessed the recoveries of diabetics using the new drug were reluctant to recommend it to their patients solely on the basis of news reports and anecdotes from the first survivors. Thousands more diabetics died because they didn't hear about insulin in time, or they didn't realize that what would happen if insulin was not taken was of greater consequence than what would happen if it was; they didn't have enough information to know that insulin was the lower-risk option. Similarly, today, diabetic people should be given information early enough in their disease process to have the option to choose a pancreas transplant before irreversible complications set in. Not giving diabetic people this information soon enough denies them their right to choose.

Until now, the medical community has been split about whether or not successful pancreas transplants actually can halt or reverse secondary complications. Some contend that without randomized clinical trials it is difficult to substantiate their success, but a number of studies published in peer-reviewed scientific journals have suggested that neuropathy, kidney disease, circulation, metabolism, and quality of life following pancreas transplants do improve. Dr. William Kennedy, a professor in the Neurology Department at the University of Minnesota, showed that following a successful pancreas transplant, nerve conduction velocity and muscle action potential improved. Only half of those people who have autonomic diabetic neuropathy survive five years, yet Dr. Kennedy shows that 85 percent of those who receive pancreas transplants are still living five years later.[8] In 1987, a German study showed increased capillary blood flow in the skin and legs of pancreas recipients.[9]

Most of us who have undergone pancreas transplants will tell you that the most important benefit is the tremendous improvement in the quality of life—improvements that go well beyond the obvious dietary flexibility and needle-free days. Hundreds of joyful anecdotes we receive at the Insulin-Free World Foundation give a personal note to the studies of post-transplant quality of life published in scientific journals.[10]

---

[8]W. R. Kennedy, X. Navarro, F. C. Goetz, D. E. R. Sutherland, and J. S. Najarian, "Effects of Pancreatic Transplantation on Diabetic Neuropathy." *New England Journal of Medicine 322,* (1990): 1031–37.

[9]D. Abendroth, V. D. Illhmer, R. Landgraf, and W. Land, "Are Late Diabetic Complications Reversible after Pancreatic Transplantation? A New Method of Follow-Up of Microcirculatory Changes." *Transplant Proceedings* 19 (1987): 2325–26.

[10]W. Piehlmeier, M. Ballinger, J. Nusser et al., "Quality of Life in Type 1 (Insulin-Independent) Diabetic Patients Prior to and after Pancreas and Kidney Transplantation in Relation to Organ Function," *Diabetologia* 34 (suppl. 1) (1991): S150–57.

It has been one and a half years since I became insulin free and I have never felt better in my life. I have started to work again and exercise every day. A life free of diabetes and insulin is truly a miracle. —*Ilya Chaus*

It's now three months post-surgery and you can't imagine how it feels to be "insulin free." It is the most incredibly, indescribable feeling. One that every diabetic deserves to know. —*Deb Kaufman*

I just spent my 18-month anniversary at Disney World. I do not ever remember having the energy level that I now enjoy. I work a good 40+ hours per week, travel for my job on occasion, am working on my master's degree and serve as a diaconate member at my church. Life is wonderful and I want to experience as much as possible. The drugs that I am required to take are just a trivial inconvenience compared to all that I went through before my transplant. —*Melodie Oesch*

Carl-Gustav Groth, M.D., Ph.D., chairman of the Department of Transplantation Surgery at the Karolinska Institute and Huddinge Hospital in Stockholm and chairman of the Nobel Assembly at the Karolinska Institute has published findings that successful pancreas transplantation can prevent a simultaneously transplanted kidney from recurrent disease.[11] The United Network for Organ Sharing, using data collected from October 1987 to June 1994, showed, convincingly, that adding a pancreas to a kidney transplant increases

[11]C. L. Zehrer and C. R. Gross, "Comparison of Quality of Life between Pancreas/Kidney and Kidney Transplant Patients: One-Year Follow-Up," *Transplant Proceedings* 26 (1994): 508–509.

the success rate for the kidney by 3 percent the first year, and by 10 percent after four years. Nevertheless, Dr. Thomas Holohan, as the director of the Office of Healthcare Technology Assessment, an office that has since been abolished, prepared a "glass-half-empty" report about pancreas transplantation for the U.S. Public Health Service in 1995[12] that influenced the financing arm of Medicare to continue denying benefits for pancreas transplants even though many commercial insurance companies list pancreas transplants as a covered benefit.

Kidney graft survival rates for diabetic kidney recipients from 10/1/87 to 6/30/94, tabulated by pancreas transplant status— simultaneous pancreas and kidney transplant (SPK) vs. kidney transplant alone (KTA)

Years post-transplant	SPK	(N)	KTA	(N)
1	83.5	(2618)	80.6	(8598)
2	78.8	(1953)	73.3	(6798)
3	74.8	(1564)	67.2	(5834)
4	70.5	(1220)	60.6	(4917)

Source: United Network for Organ Sharing Scientific Registry

In a recently published article in the *Journal of Clinical Endocrinology and Metabolism*, Dr. Holohan and Dr. Paul Robertson presented different views on whether or not pancreas transplantation has arrived as a therapeutic option for

---

[12]T. V. Holohan, "Simultaneous Pancreas-Kidney and Sequential Pancreas after Kidney Transplantation," U.S. Public Health Service, Agency for Health Care Policy and Research, Health Technology Assessment, 4:1–53.

people with insulin-dependent diabetes. Dr. Robinson writes that pancreas transplants are already being used as a therapeutic treatment for diabetic patients with kidney disease and/or uncontrollable diabetes. He approves of continued careful use of the procedure. Dr. Holohan demands a randomized clinical trial before accepting pancreas transplantation into clinical practice.

Dr. Saul Genuth, of the Division of Endocrinology at the Mount Sinai Health Care System in Cleveland, Ohio, makes an important observation in his summation of the two opinions: "Why should not individual diabetic patients receive the best treatment specific for them?"[13]

For people living with diabetes who are aware of pancreas transplantation, want options, or are faring poorly on insulin and need a pancreas transplant, Dr. Robertson's has been largely the prevailing view. Yet the ongoing controversy has led to uncertainty among many physicians about discussing pancreas transplants with their diabetic patients. Relatively few diabetic people are ever told of the option, and only 5 percent of those who could benefit actually go forward with the operation.

For diabetic individuals the question is simply this: Is there a point in the progression of diabetes where quality of life or longevity would be significantly improved by intervening with a pancreas transplant? Many diabetics go through life without having to confront any major secondary complications, but a very significant number do. As reported in sta-

[13]R. P. Robertson, T. V. Holohan, S. Genuth, "Therapeutic Controversy," *Journal of Clinical Endocrinology and Metabolism* 83, no. 6 (1998): 1872.

tistics from the National Institute of Diabetes and Digestive and Kidney Diseases and the American Academy of Ophthalmology, 30 percent progress to kidney failure, 60 percent are affected by neuropathy, and after fifteen years 80 percent develop some degree of retinopathy.[14] In those who develop diabetes as young children, these problems occur in the late twenties and thirties. The biggest problem for people trying to decide whether or not to have a pancreas transplant is that there is no way of knowing if, or when, irreversible complications may develop. Of course, it is important for people to be optimistic that they will avoid secondary complications, but for many, health unravels quickly once secondary complications do set in. It is important to have a contingency plan ready before this happens—not just a hope, but a plan formed within a framework of the evolution of new treatments and the progression of diabetes.

Until there is a way to determine who is predisposed to secondary diabetic complications, the choice between pancreas transplantation and traditional diabetes management is largely based on the *perception* of the comparative risk and reward of the two approaches. It is also influenced by expectations of how quickly diabetes research will lead to better treatments. Both pancreas transplantation *and* diabetes require long-term medical management. Ultimately each individual must choose between the side effects of immunosuppression drugs—a 1 percent incidence of skin cancer and lymphoma, an increased incidence of osteoporosis and certain infections, and cosmetic changes such as a rounded face and

[14]Statistics from American Academy of Opthalmology, 1995, educational brochure; *National Diabetes Fact Sheet*.

excess hair growth—and the risks of secondary diabetic complications.

The perception of the risks of continuing with traditional diabetes management changes as diabetes evolves from a *condition* to a *disease* and then to a *disability*. When diabetes is still a condition, the risks of secondary complications seem relatively low compared with those of immunosuppression. If diabetes progresses to the disease phase and to the early stages of complications, then people with diabetes already know they have a propensity for complications. At the Insulin-Free World Foundation, we receive most of our inquiries about pancreas transplantation from people in this last group—those who have already developed mild to severe secondary complications. There are more than 150 pancreas transplant centers in the United States, and approximately fifty more outside the U.S. Each center has its own selection criteria for transplant candidates, post-transplant protocols, and financial policies. It is important for each individual to find the right transplant center to meet his or her needs.

People who develop kidney disease need to have a realistic understanding of their treatment options: dialysis, kidney transplant alone, kidney transplant followed by a pancreas transplant, or a simultaneous pancreas and kidney transplant. Insulin injections, pumps, glucose monitoring, and diets are no match for the chaos introduced into the diabetes-management formula by dialysis, kidney transplantation, and neuropathy. Most people with insulin-dependent diabetes never have clinically significant kidney disease, but for the 30 percent who do, kidney lesions, areas of serious injury and abnormal changes, develop slowly and over a long time. These lesions progress for at least ten years after a diagnosis of diabetes before they cause any symptoms.

When given the option, most diabetic people who need a kidney transplant choose to have a pancreas transplant as well since they will have to take immunosuppression drugs for the kidney. Adding a pancreas has the added benefit of preventing the recurrence of diabetic kidney disease. As the *American Journal of Kidney Disease* reported: "Because of its ability to achieve tight glucose control, pancreas transplantation is the most effective treatment option for kidney failure resulting from insulin-dependent diabetes mellitus."[15] More than 30 percent of all institutions performing kidney transplants give their diabetic patients the option of receiving a pancreas transplant. But because most diabetic people are never told of the option, only about 40 percent of the cadaver kidneys donated to diabetic patients in the U.S. in the past few years have been transplanted in conjunction with pancreases.

In July 1998 an article published in the *New England Journal of Medicine* provided compelling data that a successful pancreas transplant does reverse secondary complications of diabetes. Dr. Michael Mauer and his colleagues at the University of Minnesota studied the kidneys of eight patients who received pancreas transplants alone, even though at the time of their transplants they had mild to advanced kidney lesions from nephropathy. Kidney biopsies were taken before the pancreas transplants were performed, then again five and

---

[15]V. Douzdjian, J. C. Rice, K. K. Gugliuzza, J. C. Fish, and R. W. Carson. "Renal Allograft and Patient Outcome after Transplantation: Pancreas-Kidney versus Kidney-Alone Transplants in Type 1 Diabetes Patients versus Kidney-Alone Transplants in Nondiabetic Patients." *American Journal of Kidney Diseases* 27, no. 1 (1996): 106–16.

ten years later. The findings were truly surprising. After ten years, the kidney lesions had actually reversed. The authors concluded that kidney lesions characteristic of diabetes are reversible with the long-term normal blood-sugar levels achieved with pancreas transplants.[16] Comparisons of long-term survival of kidney-pancreas recipients relative to diabetic recipients of kidney transplants alone from a number of transplant centers show a pronounced benefit for people who receive a pancreas in addition to a kidney. An analysis by doctor Hans Sollinger and his team at the University of Wisconsin shows that diabetic recipients of cadaver kidney transplants have an annual mortality rate of 6.2 percent and diabetic recipients of living related kidneys have an annual mortality rate of 3.65 percent. The annual mortality rate of similarly aged diabetic patients who received kidney-pancreas transplant was 1.5 percent, less than half of that of recipients of living related kidneys alone, and less than a fourth of the death rate for diabetic recipients of cadaver kidney transplants alone. Doctors Tibell and Solders and others at the Karolinska Institute in Stockholm reported that 86 percent of the recipients of kidney-pancreas transplants studied were still alive eight years after transplantation; only 47 percent of the diabetic recipients of kidney transplants alone survived eight years.[17]

[16]P. Fioretto, M. Steffes, D. E. R. Sutherland, F. Goetz, and M. Mauer, "Reversal of Lesions of Diabetic Nephropathy after Pancreas Transplantation," *New England Journal of Medicine* 339, no. 2 (1998): 69–75.

[17]A. Tibell, G. Solders, M. Larsson, C. Brattstrom, and G. Tyden, "Superior Survival after Simultaneous Pancreas and Kidney Transplantation Compared with Transplantation of a Kidney Alone in Diabetic Recipients Followed for 8 Years." *Transplant Proceedings* 29 (1–2) (1997): 668.

The accumulation of evidence that the normal blood-sugar levels achieved with pancreas transplantation do indeed reverse diabetic complications and increase life expectancy, coupled with the availability of less toxic immunosuppression protocols, will lead to more people choosing to intervene earlier in the disease process of diabetes. For the past thirty years, immunologists have studied a class of white blood cells called T-lymphocytes or T-cells responsible for the rejection of transplanted organs. Current immunosuppression drugs indiscriminately inhibit the activation of T-cells to prevent their attack on transplanted organs, but that also means their ability to attack viruses and bacteria is compromised. T-cell activation requires two signals: the first signal recognizes the target, and the second signal stimulates the T-cells to attack. In the early 1990s, agents were developed that can block the action of specific co-stimulatory agents (the second signal) to reeducate the immune system to accept transplanted tissue. These "co-stimulatory blocking reagents" have been shown to prevent the rejection of pancreas and islet transplants in large animals without impairing the immune system in general.

Decreasing the risks of transplantation by introducing less toxic immunosuppression drugs may tip the perception of risk in favor of transplantation over diabetes. Increasingly, it will be logical to offer transplants before complications of diabetes set in. Even with today's immunosuppression drugs, using pancreas transplantation to prevent diabetic kidney failure will likely become a standard treatment.

The allocation of organs in the United States is determined by computer through a priority scheme developed by United Network for Organ Sharing (UNOS), the organization that has the contract with the Department of Health and Human

Services to establish the guidelines for organ allocation. As UNOS adjusts its allocation guidelines to provide the most equitable distribution of scarce donor organs, there is an increasing urgency for people with diabetes to plan ahead. Currently, approximately five thousand donor pancreases are available for transplant per year. As discussed earlier, despite the benefits of pancreas transplantation, approximately twelve hundred donated pancreases are being used annually. Conversely, forty thousand men and women are registered on the UNOS waiting list for cadaver kidneys; only one third will receive kidneys each year, and the list is growing longer. A diabetic's chance of surviving for two years on dialysis is less than 50 percent. Few survive for more than five years. It is important for diabetic people who are concerned about kidney disease to know if they have a living donor or what they can expect on the cadaver organ waiting list should the need arise. Confronting these issues when the clock is already ticking can cause great anxiety, as one of the people in the Insulin-Free World Foundation's network wrote to us:

> There was a small discussion in last week's edition of *Parade Magazine* that gave statistics on survival rates for kidney transplant patients who had been on dialysis for 3 or more years. The rate was an alarming 44% survival. My step-daughter is on dialysis *now*. She is trying for a dual pancreas kidney transplant with a wait of about 3 years. Her brother has offered a kidney so now we are trying to assess the risk/reward benefit to her and also to her brother.

Transplant candidates can be added to the kidney waiting list at their doctor's discretion, but they cannot accumulate waiting time until their creatinine clearance, the amount of an end product of metabolism that is "cleared" by the kidneys, has fallen from a normal of approximately one hundred milliliters per minute to less than twenty milliliters per minute. By that time dialysis is generally less than a year away. Waiting time for a kidney alone varies but, on average, is about three years. The wait for a kidney *and* pancreas combined differs from one pancreas transplant center to another, depending on organ donation rates in the region and the ratio of kidney to kidney-pancreas programs that are served by each organ procurement organization (OPO). When a matching pancreas becomes available for someone waiting for a kidney and a pancreas, one of the donor's two kidneys will often be offered with the pancreas so that the kidney-pancreas transplant can be performed as a single procedure. The scarcity of kidneys is indeed an important consideration in planning a course to avoid kidney failure. Dr. Mauer's work, referred to earlier, shows that people with a predisposition for diabetic kidney disease may rescue their native kidneys by getting a solitary pancreas transplant before the deterioration becomes irreversible.

A few years after I was freed of diabetes with a successful pancreas transplant, I went back to the Joslin Diabetes Center for an eye exam. The discharge notes from earlier admissions there had tracked my progressive decline from condition to disease and on toward disability. When I returned to Joslin with my fully functional pancreas controlling my blood sugar in a nondiabetic state, I had an epiphany about the history of treatments for diabetes.

On the wall in the downstairs lobby of the magnificent new glass and steel building was a gallery of "before" and "after" black-and-white photographs of some of the first patients Dr. Joslin treated with insulin in the 1920s. As I sat in the waiting room of the eye clinic, I looked through the glass wall at a picture of a little girl in a white dress injecting insulin with a glass syringe, just as I had done when I was her age. Since then disposable plastic syringes and insulin pumps had replaced glass syringes; glucose testing using blood had replaced urine testing; laser surgery had reduced the risk of blindness, and Joslin itself had a new look and feel. But I was struck by how little the quality of life for people with diabetes had changed. Diabetics still suffer from the long-term diseases of diabetes, and they still struggle to control their blood-sugar levels.

I thought sadly about what would happen to the people in the waiting room with their squinting, glassy, unfocused, and even blinded or missing eyes as they put Band-Aids on the wounds of diabetes. I wondered if perhaps they had been told, as I was told recently in a letter from a world-renowned diabetologist, "intensive [insulin] therapy is the only hope for patients with Type 1 diabetes." Perhaps they perceived the risks of pancreas transplantation as too high and were waiting for a safer cure. Looking back at the picture on the wall I wondered how the little girl in the white dress had fared after reaching for insulin, the next medical frontier in her day. And I wondered how I would fare over the long term as a pancreas recipient. I wondered if it would be this or the next wave of science that would carry me safely into old age.

Chapter 14

Islet Transplantation

She brought me my hat, and I knew I was going out into the warm sunshine. This thought, if a wordless sensation may be called a thought, made me hop and skip with pleasure.

We walked down the path to the well-house, attracted by the fragrance of the honeysuckle with which it was covered. Someone was drawing water and my teacher placed my hand under the spout. As the cool stream gushed over my hand she spelled the word *water*, first slowly, then rapidly. I stood still, my whole attention fixed upon the motion of her fingers. Suddenly I felt a misty consciousness as of something forgotten—a thrill of returning thought; and somehow the mystery of language was revealed to me.

—*Helen Keller*, The Story of My Life

The ferocious Minnesota winter had come and gone, but its shadow hovered in the chill day. It was late March 1997 in Minneapolis, where I had been invited to speak at a reception for the Diabetes Institute for Immunology and Transplantation. It had been two and a half years since my transplant, and only the surgical scars and a limp marked me as someone who had been a patient. My work with the Insulin-Free World Foundation had taken me behind the scenes of a patient's life with diabetes to find some understanding of the science that gives us hope. I was fascinated by this world of discovery, a world of adventurers reaching across frontiers of knowledge for new insights into diabetes. Dr. David Sutherland, the director of the Diabetes Institute and the surgeon who freed me from diabetes, and Dr. Bernhard Hering, the director of the institute's islet program are now my colleagues, mentors, and friends. I go to Minneapolis often to learn from them about developments in whole-organ and cellular transplantation for diabetes, and to support the important work being undertaken there to develop a safe cure for all diabetic people.

Before my pancreas transplant my biggest fears were of being disabled by diabetes or of being stranded half-alive at thirty-something. Today my biggest fear is that my transplanted pancreas might fail. I would become diabetic again, returning to that box where my life was dictated by my metabolism. As I meet with diabetes researchers around the world to gather information for those who live from day to day with diabetes, I know that I too am looking for comfort, anxious for new options that could free me of the need for immunosuppression.

It was good to be back in Minneapolis. I felt the excitement of being among doctors and researchers who are at the forefront of the drive to cure diabetes. Dr. Sutherland had left a message at the hotel inviting me to sit in on a weekly lab meeting to be held that afternoon in one of the older hospital buildings. After checking in I hurried over to the meeting in the small conference room, which was only just big enough to accommodate the table and ten chairs. On the wall at one end of the room was a slightly torn, canvas screen reflecting a frame of light beaming up from a projector propped up on the table by a notebook and an eraser. Seated around the table were four research fellows dressed in jeans, sweaters, flannel shirts, and sneakers. They tossed me a friendly "Hi, Deb," that I knew would be the end of the small talk for the next few hours.

Dr. Sutherland came in, and the meeting began. Dr. Charlie Mills, one of the investigators, started by presenting his findings on the behavior and role of nitric oxide during islet transplantation. Although his subject might be considered of minuscule and obscure importance to the layperson, it is a matter of consequence to curing diabetes, because nitric oxide is thought to play a damaging role in islet transplantation. As Dr. Mills outlined his findings, he was stopped frequently by questions about his assumptions, the controls he used, and comparisons with earlier experiments. The group designed new experiments to be conducted the following week to try to answer some of the questions that had been raised.

Next, a visiting Japanese research fellow put a transparency on the projector and, in heavily accented English, presented his work on pancreas and islet preservation. His work was building on that of Dr. Folkert Belzer. Dr. Belzer's development of UW solution, named for the University of Wisconsin where he was the chairman of the Department of Surgery, had made it possible to preserve organs so they could be transported across the country or held until the surgeons and recipients were ready for surgery. My thoughts drifted back to a story Dr. Belzer related in Paul Terasaki's *History of Transplantation: Thirty-Five Recollections.* He recalls the path of discovery that he forged in organ preservation, describing the first clinical trial with a miniaturized version of the organ preservation machine he developed:

The opportunity arose over Christmas in 1971. We had harvested two type-A kidneys, but only one had a suitable recipient at that time. I called my good friend, Hans Dicke, a transplant surgeon in Leiden, The Netherlands, and found that they had a suitable recipient for the remaining kidney. I took the next flight from San Francisco to New York and transferred to the night flight to Amsterdam. I obtained a first class ticket to be sure to have sufficient room for the portable machine. It was Christmas Eve and the first class compartment in the 747 jet was empty except for one other passenger. Thus, I had the undivided attention of five stewardesses who kept bringing ice to keep the kidney cold. I vividly remember the Captain coming down to view the kidney and the preservation unit. He remarked how amazingly science had progressed. Here we were, flying at 30,000 feet at over 600 miles per hour in a remarkable and complex airplane, and here was a little homemade plastic box carrying, indeed, a very precious cargo. After 37 hours of preservation the kidney was successfully transplanted in a 42-year-old truck driver with polycystic kidney disease.[1]

Sitting in the unpretentious environs behind the scenes in Minnesota, and listening to the young Japanese doctor explain how he had dramatically increased preservation time for pancreases and islets by suspending them between UW and another solution, I was struck by how logically science advances. Dr. Belzer had made it possible to ship whole organs for transplantation. Now, building on his work, the

[1]F. Belzer, "Organ Preservation: A Personal Perspective," in *History of Transplantation: Thirty-Five Recollections*, ed. P. Terasaki (Los Angeles: UCLA Tissue Typing Laboratory, 1991): 601–602.

young research fellow had made it possible to preserve islet cells to ship from specialized islet isolation centers to other research labs experimenting with them.

The data that were presented had been corroborated by a series of experiments with consistent results. Furthermore, Dr. Sutherland could find no flaws in the design of the experiments or in any of the conclusions that had been reached. Without further ado he recommended that an abstract be submitted to the American Society of Transplant Surgeons to undergo peer review, and that the new preservation method be used clinically as soon as possible. Dr. Sutherland smiled in his small-town, boy-next-door way, waved a waist-high, vintage Sutherland wave with his left hand and started for the door. Deferentially, the young doctor called after him.

"Ah, excuse me, Dr. Sutherland?"

"Yes?" he said from the door.

"I have to tell you," the young doctor said somewhat apologetically and at the same time amused. "I am using a Japanese pickle machine for my preservation chamber!"

The unassuming humanity of Dr. Belzer's tale in light of the tremendous advances in transplantation that it produced, and the creative spirit that had inspired the use of a pickle machine to preserve organs, illustrate that science is advanced by acts of human will. Indeed, it is unlikely that there will be a "Eureka" moment when *a* cure, *the* cure, the one time, forever antidote to diabetes is discovered. Cures evolve. Pancreas transplantation evolved from a long era of "treatments," and it has paved the way for a new era of "cures." Clearly, pancreas transplantation is not a perfect cure; because of its inherent surgical and immunological risks, it is rarely applied early enough in the disease process of individuals to eliminate secondary complications.

But what if normal glucose metabolism could be reinstated in every diabetic, newly diagnosed or veteran, for a lifetime, with a single injection of cells and without the need for immunosuppression drugs? Less than a thimbleful of islet cells, about 1 cc, is all that is needed to restore normal blood-sugar levels in people with insulin-dependent diabetes, yet today the only consistently successful way to transplant them is as part of a whole pancreas organ.

The islets account for a mere 1 to 2 percent of the pancreas. The rest of the organ is made up of the exocrine tissue. Ironically, it is the ongoing drainage of 1 to 1.5 liters of digestive enzymes per day from the exocrine tissue that causes most of the surgical complications with pancreas transplants. The exocrine portion of the pancreas functions normally in diabetic people, so the transplanted pancreas is attached to the bladder or intestine to drain its secretions, whereas normally a pancreas drains into the stomach. If the drainage gets blocked, then the pancreas can become inflamed or infected, causing pancreatitis. It has been a dream since the early 1960s that transplanting just the insulin-producing cells could achieve the same results as pancreas transplantation while virtually eliminating the surgical risk. If this could be achieved, and if the immune system could be modified specifically to tolerate transplanted islet cells so that long-term immunosuppression agents could be discontinued or reduced, then whole-pancreas transplants would be obsolete. More diabetic people and their medical advisors would choose to intervene *before* the secondary complications of diabetes are manifest.

Islets, the "little heap of cells" that had no more than a walk-on part when Paul Langerhans discovered them more than 120 years ago, play a leading role today in the final act of the era of insulin. The islets house an extremely complex and sensitive mechanism for spontaneously regulating the production of insulin and glucagon with exquisite accuracy. A single pancreas contains 1 to 1.5 million islets. Each islet is made up of about 2,500 cells, the majority of which are the insulin-producing beta cells. Transplanting these tiny clusters of islets, however, has proven to be a very big challenge. The first person to make any significant headway was Dr. Paul Lacy. In the late 1960s at Washington University in St. Louis, he achieved some very promising results in small rodents. In 1972 Dr. Lacy co-authored an article with Dr. Walter Ballinger that was published in *Surgery* and titled, "Transplantation of Intact Pancreatic Islets in Rats."[2] In this seminal article in islet transplantation, the two scientists reported that they had cured diabetes in rodents by transplanting islets that had been isolated from the pancreas. This was such an exciting and relatively easy success that many believed there would be a human cure using islets in a few years. Yet, even as thousands of researchers around the world have picked up the banner and pursued the dream from a variety of different angles, it seems that more questions than answers have been uncovered. Still there has been much progress.

Doctors John Najarian and David Sutherland performed

[2]W. F. Ballinger and P. E. Lacy, "Transplantation of Intact Pancreatic Islets in Rats," *Surgery* 72 (1972): 175–86.

the first series of ten islet transplant procedures in seven diabetic people at the University of Minnesota from 1974 to
1977, but none of the recipients had any measurable increase
in insulin production.[3] It wasn't until 1989 that an islet transplant performed by Dr. Lacy and Dr. David Scharp at Washington University actually rendered a diabetic recipient
insulin independent.[4] The islets were injected into the
patient's portal vein, where the force of the blood flow
lodged them in the small capillaries in the liver and they
became part of the vascular system. Incredibly, the whole
procedure took approximately thirty minutes and was done
under local anesthesia.

From 1974 to 1996, 305 islet transplants were performed
worldwide on people with insulin-dependent diabetes.
Thirty-five (11 percent) of the recipients became insulin
independent for periods ranging from thirteen days to more
than five and a half years. The average duration of insulin
independence was approximately fifteen months. Although
most recipients had to resume insulin regimens, the islet
transplants did result in more stable blood-sugar control
using less insulin and, most important, the absence of severe
hypoglycemia. Furthermore, the fact that in some instances
the transplanted islets were capable of normalizing blood-
sugar levels of Type 1 diabetics without the need for exogenous insulin leaves no doubt that insulin independence is

[3]J. S. Najarian, D. E. R. Sutherland, A. J. Matas et al., "Human Islet
Transplantation: A Preliminary Report," *Transplantation Proceedings* 9,
no 1 (1977): 233–36.

[4]D. W. Scharp, P. E. Lacy, J. V. Santiago, C. S. McCullough et. al.,
"Insulin Independence after Islet Transplantation into Type 1 Diabetic
Patients," *Diabetes* 39 (1990): 515–18.

possible with islet transplants. Now the question is, Which variables lead to success, and what are the mechanisms of failure?

The failures have been attributed broadly to three areas:

- Too few islets "engrafting," being viable, after transplantation to sustain a nondiabetic state.
- Immune-mediated destruction caused by, for example, the islets being damaged by a general inflammatory response soon after the donor islets are introduced to the recipient, or later when classic rejection destroys the islets. Similarly, an *auto*immune attack can kill the insulin-producing beta cells and cause the recurrence of diabetes.
- The toxic effect of diabetogenic immunosuppression drugs—drugs used to prevent rejection that have the side effect of causing diabetes.

Reviewing the islet transplant successes so far shows a strong correlation between the number of islets that are transplanted and subsequent outcomes for the recipients. The best clinical results have been achieved when for each kilogram (2.2 pounds) the recipient weighs, at least 6,000 islets and as many as several million (with a mean of 12,300 islets) have been transplanted. Therefore, one of the first challenges to overcome in islet transplantation was to optimize the number of islets being transplanted by learning how to isolate them from the surrounding exocrine tissue without damaging them in the process.

In 1988, while working with doctors Lacy and Scharp at Washington University, Dr. Camillo Ricordi surmounted this obstacle. Dr. Ricordi, who is now the scientific director and chief academic officer of the Diabetes Research Institute at the University of Miami Medical School, perfected an automated method of isolating islets that made it possible, for the first time, to retrieve enough human islets from a *single* donor pancreas to reverse diabetes. The development of this method led to the first series of prolonged insulin independence, with seven out of nine islet recipients at the Diabetes Research Institute in Miami remaining insulin free for up to five years. Other islet centers, including the University of Alberta Hospital in Edmonton, the Instituto San Raffaele Hospital in Milan, and the University of Minnesota in Minneapolis began to see successes using this new automated method of isolating islets. Today, 95 percent of the world's transplant centers conducting human islet trials use Dr. Ricordi's automated islet isolation technique, aptly called the "Ricordi chamber."

The yield of islets that can be isolated from a single pancreas has been further enhanced by improvements in the quality of collagenase, the blend of digestive enzymes used to break down the exocrine tissue of the pancreas to release the islets. Not only are these significant achievements in terms of helping to address the anticipated scarcity of donor pancreases, they may provide immunological advantages by simplifying tissue matching to a single donor source, rather than to the multiple tissue types present when several pancreases are required.

To gauge progress in islet transplantation, it is important to take a more granular measure of improvement than to apply the ultimate standard of insulin independence that is used to define success with pancreas transplants. One marker used to measure success with islet transplants is the production of C-peptide. Measurable amounts of C-peptide in the blood indicates insulin production and consequently islet function. The most consistent success with human islet transplants so far was recorded in a series of twelve procedures done in Giessen, Germany, by doctors Bernhard Hering and Reinhard Bretzel. In this series, 100 percent of the islet recipients were still showing C-peptide production three months after transplantation. One-third of them were completely insulin independent at one year, and 45 percent of the recipients maintained superior metabolic control to that which can be achieved with exogenous insulin. The longest-functioning islet transplant to date was performed by Dr. Rodolfo Alejandro at the University of Miami in the early 1990s, with the islets functioning for more than seven years.[5] Even though the islet recipients continued to require insulin, the amount of insulin secreted was adequate to maintain normal glucose levels—without hypoglycemia—something that was not possible with intensive insulin therapy as practiced in the DCCT.

So far, even a full complement of healthy islets has not achieved the consistent success rates of whole-organ pancreas transplants because free-floating islets are more vulnerable to attack from the immune system. Transplanting cells to treat a range of human diseases has been limited because of the swift destruction by the recipient's immune system. One idea being researched is to isolate transplanted cells from the immune system altogether by first enclosing them in a semipermeable membrane, a process known as immunoisolation. In the case of transplanting human islets, ideally the membrane would protect the encapsulated islets from the diffuse and complex network of interacting cells and tissues that make up the immune system, while at the same time allowing the elements required to stimulate insulin secretion to pass

---

[5] R. Alejandro, R. Lehmann, C. Ricordi, et. al., "Long-term Function (Six Years) of Islet Allografts in Diabetes," *Diabetes* 46 (1997): 1983–89.

through. In addition, immunoisolation devices have to allow entry to oxygen and other nutrients to keep the encapsulated cells alive and healthy.

Scientists in industry and academia have engineered a wide variety of devices in their search for effective technologies to encapsulate islets: tubular membranes, flat sandwich pouches, microcapsules (which encapsulate cells individually), macro-capsules (which encapsulate many cells in a single device), hollow fibers, and intravascular devices.[6] There have been advances with encapsulation; a few companies have shown that encapsulation can work when encapsulated pig islets are transplanted into dogs. Because much of the work with encapsulation in industry is veiled in corporate secrecy, it may be that the successes and failures extend beyond what the public has been told.

Nonetheless, problems with encapsulation remain. The functioning of the devices can become impaired by fibrosis (growth of scar tissue). Also, the capsule size needed to contain the volume of islets necessary to normalize blood-sugar levels, and enough space to maintain the viability of the islets inside, is impractically large. The limited trials in transplanting encapsulated islets into humans that have been done required islets from five to eight pancreases to overcome the restricted exchange of insulin and glucose across the capsule membrane(s). Unfortunately, recipients of encapsulated islets haven't been freed of either the need to take immunosuppression drugs *or* insulin post-transplant, whereas pancreas recipients and a few of the recipients of free-floating islets have been freed of the need to take insulin.

---

[6]T. Wang, I. Lacik et al., "An Encapsulation System for the Immuno-isolation of Pancreatic Islets," *Nature Biotechnology* 15 (1997): 358–62.

Given that 80 percent of the time, a single pancreas transplanted as a whole organ can provide complete insulin independence, the use of multiple donors for a single islet transplant will be increasingly difficult to justify as the demand for pancreases approaches the supply. The need for a large number of cells, however, does not itself imply the failure of encapsulation technologies. Indeed, encapsulation may play a very important role when it is possible to engineer cell lines (self-perpetuating strings of cells) to create an inexhaustible supply of insulin-producing cells. Nevertheless, in the short term human pancreases are available for islet transplant experiments and should be used to learn about surgical technique, islet placement in the body, monitoring of rejection, salvaging transplanted islets, and autoimmunity.

The most striking success story with islet transplantation is that of Don Smith, who, after thirty years with insulin-dependent diabetes, made history by remaining insulin free for more than five and a half years after receiving 1.3 million islets in a St. Louis operating room. Dr. Lacy and Dr. Scharp directed the procedure. Don embodies the dream of islet transplantation. Last May, speaking to more than four hundred people at the Insulin-Free World Foundation's seminar in St. Louis, Don exclaimed, "I lived, when according to the statistics I should be dead!"

Islet transplants can already benefit people who suffer from severe hypoglycemia or persistently labile (uncontrollable) diabetes. But if islet transplantation is to replace pancreas transplantation, it must be a consistently successful means of becoming insulin free. It must also be possible without the need for immunosuppression drugs. Dr. Starzl's comment that immunosuppression is the "heart and soul and philosophy" of transplantation certainly seems to be the case with transplanting fragile cells, which are more susceptible to both immune and autoimmune attacks than are whole organs.

The steroid- and Cyclosporine-based immunosuppression regimens that work well with whole organ transplantation have diabetogenic side effects that place an undue burden on newly transplanted cells. In the last two or three years a limited number of clinical trials using immunosuppression protocols designed specifically for islet transplants have begun to achieve more consistent success. "In the past, people doing islet transplants were using protocols designed for whole-organ transplantation," says Dr. Hering, "and these were insufficient to cope with the special complexities of islet transplantation. And what's more, many more tools are available that are bringing us closer in our quest for methods of achieving immunological tolerance in islet transplantation"— the acceptance of foreign tissue without the need for lifelong immunosuppression.

The recent development of co-stimulatory blocking agents—the new class of drugs that may make it possible to reeducate the immune system to accept foreign tissue (mentioned in the last chapter)—has excited the islet research community. When used alone or in combination with other drugs, they have successfully prevented the rejection of transplanted islets in monkeys while leaving the animals insulin free and without any apparent harm to their immune systems. The first ground-breaking results came from studies conducted by Captain David M. Harlan, Commander Allan Kirk, and Dr. Tom Davis of the United States Navy Medical Corps, in collaboration with doctors Stuart Knechtle and John Fechner at the University of Wisconsin.

Describing their work in *Proceedings of the National Academy of Sciences*,[7] the investigators reported that rhesus monkeys implanted with mismatched kidneys and receiving co-stimulatory blocking agents not only tolerated the medicines without any toxicity, but had no episodes of rejection for at least six months following the transplant. The new co-stimulatory blocking agents did not show "diabetogenic" side effects; indeed, they even seem to have the potential to inhibit inflammation after surgery. In islet transplants, this often-recurring response limits the number of islets that survive transplantation.

To further this success, the Diabetes Research Institute in Miami embarked on a series of preclinical trials under the direction of doctors Camillo Ricordi and Norma Kenyon, using a co-stimulatory blocking agent known as anti-CD154 by itself in primates. Again, rejection was prevented, and the diabetic monkeys who received islet transplants sustained insulin independence. Co-stimulatory blocking agents are "the most promising thing that has come around for a long time," says Dr. Hering of the Diabetes Institute for Immunology and Transplantation at the University of Minnesota. "There's an endless list of protocols that work in mice and rats," he points out, "but in primates, there's been nothing. In contrast, the metabolic outcomes here are spectacular. The animals were perfectly normoglycemic." However, Dr. Hering and others are quick to acknowledge that much work remains to be done. "These studies need to be repeated and extended

[7] A. Kirk, D. Harlan, N. Armstrong, T. Davis et al., "CTLA4-Ig and Anti-CD40 Ligand Prevent Renal Allograft Rejection in Primates," *Proceedings of the National Academy of Sciences* 94 (1997): 8789–94.

in additional animal studies," says Captain Harlan, "and the therapy needs to be studied in carefully designed human trials. If preliminary results hold, however, then perhaps a new era in transplantation medicine may be on the horizon."[8]

Dr. Kenyon drew a graph that makes a most striking visual statement about how imminently beneficial these findings could be. The soon-to-be-published graph shows postprandial blood-sugar levels of formerly diabetic monkey islet recipients that are free of the need for both insulin and ongoing immunosuppression therapy. The data points form a steady line depicting consistently normal blood-sugar levels. Dr. Kenyon superimposed this graph on a graph she made of her young diabetic daughter's blood-sugar levels after eating. Her daughter practices intensive insulin therapy and is considered to have good blood-sugar control, yet the data points form a line that swings from peaks to troughs around the targeted blood-sugar range. One is left with the impression that islet transplantation in humans, without the need for ongoing immunosuppression, is scientifically possible.

The demand for donor human pancreases for whole organ and islet transplants will continue to escalate, yet there will be too few to keep up with the new cases of diabetes being diagnosed and to take care of those people who already have diabetes. For islet or pancreas therapy to have a significant impact on the human and economic toll exacted by diabetes, a reproducible and inexhaustible supply of pancreases, islets, or insulin-producing cells needs to be established. The very fact that islets are islets, that they are discrete cells, means they can

[8]M. Burton, "The Time is Now," *Insulin-Free*TIMES (Summer 1998): 6.

be isolated, manipulated, and reproduced. Unlike whole or partial pancreases, islets have the potential to cater to the demand of millions of diabetic people. Diabetes researchers are studying a variety of sources for cell-based insulin replacement. With the momentum of research and clinical experience that has been building in transplanting islets, islet transplantation will explode into the forefront of treatments for diabetes when any one of the alternative sources of islets being researched becomes a viable option. Five alternative sources of insulin-producing cells are currently being investigated:

- Xenogeneic cells—cells from another species
- Expanded adult or fetal human beta cells
- Engineered cell lines—genetically manipulated strings of self-perpetuating cells
- Immortalized cell lines—naturally replicating cells from malignant tumors
- Proliferated or regenerated cells from a person's native islets

For some time, transplanting tissues or cells from animals into humans has been thought of as a possible solution for end-stage organ failure. For a brief moment in the early 1960s, dialysis was not successful and people who died of brain death were not yet accepted as donors, so only transplants from well-matched living donors were possible. There were no treatments for people who were dying of kidney failure and who did not have living donors with a closely matched tissue type. During this fallow time in treatments, a forty-three-year-old dock worker named Jefferson Davis was dying of kidney failure and had no family donor. It was in this environment that Dr. Keith Reemtsma, a transplant surgeon at Tulane University Hospital in New Orleans, performed an unimaginable procedure to try to save Jefferson Davis. In December of 1963 he transplanted the kidneys of a chimpanzee into his patient. What is even more remarkable is that the "xenograft"—the scientific term denoting organs, tissue, or cells taken from one species and transplanted into another—functioned normally for nine weeks before Jefferson Davis died of septic shock. An autopsy revealed normal function in the transplanted kidneys with no signs of rejection. The following month, Dr. Reemtsma did another xenotransplant for a patient who survived for nine *months.* By 1965 dialysis and kidney transplants using cadaveric donors were possible treatments, so xenotransplantation experiments were discontinued.

During the past decade, however, the limitations imposed by the shortage of human-cadaver donor organs on the field of transplantation in general has rekindled the concept of xenotransplantation. At the same time, advances in immunology and the understanding of the mechanisms of tissue rejection make it reasonable to believe that xenogeneic cells and tissues can be engineered to prevent rejection. For a variety of reasons—some scientific and others ethical or philosophical—pigs are viewed as a promising species to provide islets in sufficient quantities to treat the millions of diabetic people. Pig and human islets have similar setpoints, the glucose level in the blood at which the islets secrete insulin. The structures of pig and human insulins differ by only one amino acid, and pigs breed quickly and have large litters. Because of the heated philosophical debate about the use of animal organs for transplantation into humans, perhaps pigs are a more publicly acceptable islet donor candidate because their pancreases have been used for years to extract insulin, their heart valves are widely used to correct cardiac problems, and they are an accepted part of the food chain for humans.

The use of pig islets for transplantation has been stalled by ongoing disagreements about xenotransplantation in general and the fear that transplanted xenogeneic tissue and cells will transmit diseases through retroviruses to humans. (For example, when viruses become part of human DNA and create new strands of "retroviruses.") Regulatory organizations and virologists, for whom the benefits of xenotransplantation are small and the perception of risk high, fall on one side of the argument. The other consists of those with life-threatening organ failure and the scientists working to find solutions for them. This debate has fluctuated from one polar extreme to the other, with moratoriums and sanctions alternately placed on the use of animal tissue in humans. Both sides agree, however, that xenotransplantation needs to be approached thoughtfully and with caution; the controversy arises over how quickly human studies should progress.

From 1990 to 1993, before there were any regulations to the contrary, Dr. Carl Groth, a pioneer and leader in the field of pancreas and islet transplantation and professor of transplantation surgery at the Karolinska Institute in Stockholm, directed a clinical pilot study in which fetal pig islet cell clusters were transplanted into ten human diabetic patients. Small traces of porcine C-peptide were detected in the urine of four of the recipients, showing that there had been some secretion of pig insulin from the transplanted islets. In fact, some pig islets that escaped rejection were found in tests performed on one patient.

In 1996 and 1997, the use of pig organs for xenotransplantation was sanctioned by the Department of Health's Advisory Group on the Ethics of Xenotransplantation in the United Kingdom by the Institute of Medicine in the United States, and again in the United Kingdom by the Nuffield Council on Bioethics—but in 1997 the tide turned again. Robin Weiss of the Institute of Cancer Research in London and David Onions at the University of Glasgow showed in culture (in a controlled laboratory setting) that two normally dormant retroviruses in the DNA of pigs could possibly become active in humans. The U.S. Food and Drug Administration promptly prohibited any pig organ transplants. In 1998, Walid Heinene and Louisa Chapman of the Center for Disease Control studied the ten Swedish patients who had received pig islets in the early 1990s. They found no trace of pig virus DNA or any antibodies to pig viruses. Nor did they find enzymes that would indicate unidentified viruses were present. "We looked in blood, lymphocytes [white blood corpuscles], and serum, and found nothing. These are reassuring data," Heinene said, and then added that the relevance of these findings beyond the small study group was unknown. While ethicists, politicians, scientists, and patients are embroiled in debating guidelines, work continues in laboratories to find yet other sources of islets.

Diabetes is one of many diseases or traumas that result from the destruction or degeneration of cells. For example, Parkinson's and Huntington's disease result from the degeneration of neurons in the brain; severe burns destroy skin cells. Cellular biologists dream of getting cells to reproduce in a controlled lab setting to provide an immortal, or limitless, supply of cells to treat and cure these diseases. For diabetes researchers, the goal is to make islet cells reproduce so that each islet multiplies into many islets. If this becomes possible, then a parent could donate, for example, a fifth of a pancreas to free his or her child of diabetes. Perhaps islets that escape the autoimmune attack that precipitates diabetes could be isolated from the pancreases of diabetic people, multiplied in test tubes, taught how to make insulin and fend off autoimmunity, and be returned to the person without provoking rejection. These are the kinds of very big objectives that characterize diabetes research today.

In September 1996, *Diabetes* reported that scientists at the islet research laboratory at The ScrippsWhittier Institute for Diabetes at the University of California, San Diego, had for the first time shown that adult human pancreatic cells can be replicated; they had achieved a thirtyfold increase in the cells.[9] By placing adult islets into structures called matrices and adding growth factors—hormonelike substances that stimulate cells to multiply—they succeeded in getting the islets to proliferate (multiply) to form "monolayers of cells," sheets of single layers of replicated cells. They also identified substances that inhibit growth. By blocking these agents, they were able to accelerate proliferation. Scientists at The ScrippsWhittier Institute are now able to expand adult human islet cells twenty to thirty *thousand*fold.

However, replicating islets is only part of a larger challenge; the new islets must also produce insulin and regulate blood-sugar levels. So far, as the cells replicate they produce

[9]G. M. Beattie, J. S. Rubin, M. I. Mally, T. Otonkiski, A. Hayek, "Regulation of Proliferation and Differentiation of Human Fetal Pancreatic Islet Cells by Extracellular Matrix, Hepatocyte Growth Factor, and Cell-Cell Contact," *Diabetes* 45 (1996): 1223–28.

less and less insulin and they senesce—die prematurely of old age. Each time the cells divide, telomeres, structures at the end of the chromosomes, shorten until ultimately they are too short to divide further. An article in the January 16, 1998, issue of *Science*, showed that when the telomerase gene is inserted into cells, the cells continue to replicate with a life span of normal human cells, indeed a significant finding.[10] Nevertheless, it's important to keep research "breakthroughs" in perspective.

Dr. Alberto Hayek, professor of pediatrics and director of the islet cell laboratories at ScrippsWhittier, says, "There have been two hundred trials with gene therapy in many diseases and none of them have worked, but that doesn't mean that it will not work one day." He continues: "We have already been able to insert the insulin gene into fetal cells, and, one day, we will be able to insert genes to prevent our immunity—so we will have, in one cell, the ability to both cure diabetes and to avoid the relapse of disease."

In a study similar to Dr. Hayek's work with beta-cell proliferation, Dr. Aaron Vinik, director of the Diabetes Research Institute at the Diabetes Institutes of Eastern Virginia Medical School, is working on the neogenesis (regeneration) and differentiation of precursor cells derived from cells in the pancreatic ducts. The entire islet mass of an adult develops in the prenatal period; after birth the cells regenerate through cell division. But the division of mature islets is slow. Dr. Vinik is working to find ways to reiterate the prenatal development of

---

[10]A. G. Bodnar, M. Ouellette, M. Frolkis, S. E. Holt et al., "Extension of Life-Span by Introduction of Telomerase into Normal Human Cells," *Science* 279 (1998): 349–52.

beta cells in laboratory animals. If autoimmunity can be overcome, it may be possible to regenerate a diabetic person's surviving beta cells to provide a large enough mass to control blood-sugar levels without the need for immunosuppression.

Dr. Christopher Newgard of the Gifford Laboratories for Diabetes Research and professor of biochemistry and internal medicine at the University of Texas Southwestern Medical Center in Dallas is working on applying genetic engineering to the development of cell lines that will provide a *replenishable, stable,* and *immunoprotected* supply of surrogate islet cells for transplantation. Not only must the engineered cells have a consistent set of traits (genotypic stability), they must each respond in precisely the same way to physiological cues (phenotypic stability). They must maintain this genotypic and phenotypic stability on a scale large enough to treat millions of diabetics with perfect consistency from lot to lot for years to come. Growing large quantities of cells without the "replicative senescence" that causes diminished insulin production is imperative to achieving this goal, but as yet no immortal human cell lines have been developed. This challenge is not unique to genetically engineered human cells; indeed, isolating large numbers of functionally equivalent pig islets has also been problematic. Until functionally stable human cell lines can be grown, Dr. Newgard and others are using existing animal cell lines to learn how to modify them to function like islet cells.

Using cell lines that naturally do not produce insulin, researchers insert (transfect) DNA into the cells to cause an overproduction of insulin; then they regulate the amount of insulin that is released by the cells in response to glucose. By experimenting with various types of cells and genetic material, they have been able to get cells to secrete insulin in response to glucose, but with a very low response rate relative to that of normal islets. Nonetheless, the fact that the cells produced insulin has proven in principle that non-insulin-producing cells can be engineered to produce and secrete insulin. Dr. Newgard and his colleagues' recent work has concentrated on using rodent insulinomas (cancer cells). Through testing a series of genes, they were able to increase insulin secretion in response to glucose six- to eightfold. Not only was this an improved insulin response over unengineered cells, but the ability of the cells to secrete insulin was sustained. The setpoint for insulin secretion has yet to be adjusted, but the genetically engineered rodent insulinoma cell lines seem to have exceptional genotypic and phenotypic stability.

For these cells to be true surrogates for islets, they need to be engineered to fend off immunity or protected from it with immunosuppression and/or encapsulation. Several strategies of immunoprotection are being studied: pretreating or engineering cells so they are not recognized by the immune system as "non-self" cells; developing a separate cell line that could provide protection and be transplanted at the same time as the "islet" cell line; or encapsulating the cells so the recipient is protected from malfunctioning cells and the cells are protected from the immune system.

Whether the islet cells are free-floating, xenogeneic, encapsulated, tolerated, expanded, regenerated, engineered—or, most likely, some combination of these approaches—islet cell transplantation is moving toward curing diabetes with substantial momentum. As Dr. Bernhard Hering, one of today's most influential contributors to islet transplantation, says, "There is a learning curve in islet transplantation, just as there was in kidney, heart, and pancreas transplantation. We have many things that have worked out, not only in mice and rats, but also in large animals. Now we have to get to the final step—implementation."

Chapter 15

The Bird Is in Your Hands

Great rivers flow with an energy created by all the seemingly unrelated and independent tributaries, springs, and rains that feed them. Such rivers not only absorb this energy, they provide purpose and direction, and with their currents carry everything in their path.

—*Thomas M. Wendel, Chairman and CEO,*
BRIDGE Information Systems

In the 1920s, polio struck quickly, crippling its victims, leaving them in iron lungs, on crutches, paralyzed, and in wheelchairs. As with diabetes, there was little knowledge about polio and how it was transmitted. Franklin Delano Roosevelt was paralyzed by polio and in a wheelchair when he was inaugurated as president of the United States in 1933. With one foot in the presidency, and one in his world of disease, FDR led the American people from 1933 to 1945, through the Great Depression, the success of the New Deal, and World War II. And, on another front, FDR waged a war against polio that, after his death, was won.

Science had shown that, in theory, vaccines could protect

against viruses, and FDR determined that he would translate that theory into a way to rid the world of polio. He established the National Foundation for Infantile Paralysis, commonly known as the March of Dimes, raised millions of dollars, and directed resources to develop a vaccine against the poliovirus. FDR saw the long-term value of using public policy and government assistance to rehabilitate people with disabilities, and often aimed tax laws and savings plans to that end. As part of the New Deal he had promised the American people during his 1932 presidential campaign, FDR introduced social security and unemployment insurance. Hospitalizations, operations, adaptive equipment, and rehabilitation were provided for polio patients, regardless of their income or insurance. And with the same charisma that FDR used to harness and direct the energies of the vast national listening audience during his trademark radio "Fireside Chats," FDR rallied public support to fight polio.

Because eradicating polio was a well-funded national priority, the challenge attracted many of the best and brightest scientists to the field, including a then recent graduate of New York University Medical School, Dr. Jonas Salk. While attending medical school, Salk had spent a year researching the recently discovered flu virus and had found a way to provide immunity to the illness. In 1947, Salk accepted an appointment to the University of Pittsburgh Medical School where he worked with the National Foundation (the March of Dimes). For eight years he devoted his time to developing a vaccine using inactive (dead) samples of the poliovirus that were injected to reeducate the immune system to defend the body against polio. Dr. Albert Sabin, at the University of Cincinnati Medical School, had also picked up the challenge and was working on a vaccine using small amounts of live poliovirus that could be taken orally. Salk and Sabin each had proponents and critics, but both of their research approaches developed into effective immunizations against polio.

Connaught Medical Research Laboratories in Toronto played a key role by procuring the monkey kidneys required to make Salk's vaccine, and by developing a way to make the vaccine safe for use in children. Through the winter of 1953 to 1954, Connaught sent bottles of vaccine from the labs in Toronto to drug companies in Detroit and Indianapolis where the processing was completed. In April, a team of researchers, led by Dr. Salk and orchestrated by the March of Dimes and Connaught Laboratories, tested the vaccine on 1.8 million children. It was the largest clinical trial in the history of medicine. A year later, Salk's polio vaccine was made public, with Salk himself holding the patent to protect the price of the new drug from rising for commercial gain. In 1954, the year the vaccine was introduced, there were 54,000 new cases of polio. Three years later, fewer than two hundred people contracted the virus. In 1985, the Pan American Health Organization (PAHO) vowed to free the Western Hemisphere of the last vestiges of the virus by 1990. Indeed, the last confirmed case was reported in 1991 in Peru. In 1988, the World Health Assembly, with strategic direction from the World Health Organization (WHO), established the objective of eradicating polio worldwide by the year 2000.[1]

Beyond the incalculable human benefit, it is estimated that

[1]World Health Assembly, *Global Eradication of Poliomyelitis by the Year 2000* (Geneva: World Health Organization, January 1995).

the reduction in health-care expenditures made possible by the polio vaccine compensates for its development costs every three weeks. But freeing the Western Hemisphere, and, it is hoped, soon the world, from polio was not possible because of science alone—it took a unified, collaborative, and focused effort on all fronts: social, political, and economic.

I recount the battle against polio because there are great similarities between overcoming that disabling virus and the challenges we face now in our showdown with diabetes. Sixteen million Americans have diabetes.[2] Every three minutes, one American dies from diabetes[3] and four are diagnosed. Diabetes costs $91.1 *billion* annually, accounting for one of every four Medicare dollars and one of every seven health-care dollars spent in the United States.[4] The direct medical cost of blindness per diabetic patient per year, based on Medicare figures, is $2,000.[5] With as many as 24,000 new cases of blindness caused by diabetes each year, costs increase by $48 million per year. Diabetes is the leading cause of kidney failure, accounting for about 40 percent of new dialysis and kidney transplant patients, approximately

---

[2]American Diabetes Association, *Diabetes Facts and Figures*, 1997.

[3]Juvenile Diabetes Foundation International, *Diabetes Facts*, 1998.

[4]R. J. Rubin, W. M. Altman, and D. N. Mendelson, "Health-Care Expenditures for People with Diabetes Mellitus," *Journal of Clinical Endocrinology and Metabolism* 78 (1992): 809.

[5]Y. P. Chiang, L. J. Bassi, and J. C. Javitt, "Federal Budgetary Costs of Blindness," *Millbank Quarterly* 70 (1992): 319–40.

30,000 people.[6] At an annual cost per patient of $45,000 for dialysis,[7] new cases of kidney failure escalate the cost of diabetes to taxpayers by more than a billion dollars per year. Sixty to 70 percent of the diabetic population has diabetic nerve damage, which, in severe forms, can lead to lower limb amputations. Diabetes is the most frequent cause of nontraumatic lower limb amputation, with a fifteen to forty times greater risk and more than 56,000 limbs lost to diabetes per year.[8] The cost per event is $29,500,[9] resulting in a $1.5 billion increase in the cost of diabetes every year. Middle-aged people with diabetes are two to four times more likely to have heart disease, which is present in 77,000 (43 percent) of diabetes-related deaths.[10] And diabetic people are two to four times more likely to have a stroke. Six percent of the population in the United States has diabetes, yet diabetes accounts for a disproportionate

[6]Centers for Disease Control and Prevention, *National Diabetes Fact Sheet: National Estimates and General Information on Diabetes in the United States* (Atlanta: U.S. Department of Health and Human Services, 1997).

[7]U. S. Renal Data System, *USRDA 1995 Annual Data Report* (Bethesda, Md.: National Institutes of Health, National Institute of Diabetes and Digestive and Kidney Diseases, April 1995).

[8]*Diabetes Facts and Figures*, 1997.

[9]M. H. Eckman, S. Greenfield, W. C. Mackey et al., "Foot Infections in Diabetic Patients: Decision and Cost-Effectiveness Analyses," *Journal of the American Medical Association* 273 (1995): 712–20.

[10]Centers for Disease Control and Prevention, *National Diabetes Fact Sheet: National Estimates and General Information on Diabetes in the United States* (Atlanta: U.S. Department of Health and Human Services, 1997).

15 percent of the total U.S. health-care budget.[11] The total annual per capita medical expenditure incurred per diabetic person per year is $10,071, compared with $2,669 for nondiabetic people.[12]

The escalating human and monetary costs of diabetes—for individuals and for society as a whole—place an excessive demand on the already overburdened health-care system. Our medical system was built around the short-term costs of

Leading causes of death, in descending order, as reported by the Centers for Disease Control and Prevention

1900	1998
pneumonia	heart disease
tuberculosis	cancer
enteritis	stroke
heart disease	chronic obstructive pulmonary diseases
vascular lesions	accidents
nephritis	pneumonia/influenza
accidents	diabetes mellitus
cancer	HIV/AIDS

Source: Centers for Disease Control and Prevention, "Ten Leading Causes of Death in the U.S. (1996, All Ages)," *Monthly Vital Statistics Report*, 46, no.1 (suppl).

[11]N. Fox-Ray, M. Thamer, E. Gardner, and J. Chan, "Economic Consequences of Diabetes Mellitus in the U.S. in 1997," *Diabetes Care* 21, no. 2 (1998): 296–309.

[12]N. Fox-Ray et al., "Economic Consequences of Diabetes Mellitus," 296.

treating accidents and catastrophic illnesses, the leading causes of death in the first part of the twentieth century. Advances in medicine have cured most of those illnesses. Today, *chronic* diseases account for 80 percent of U.S. health-care costs and are the leading causes of death.

One conceptual model of health-care utilization I heard presented at a disease-management conference for providers (hospitals, doctors, home care) and payers (insurance companies, Medicare, Medicaid) illustrated the cost of illness, injury, and disease with respect to three measures (Figure III):

Figure III: Profiles of disease.

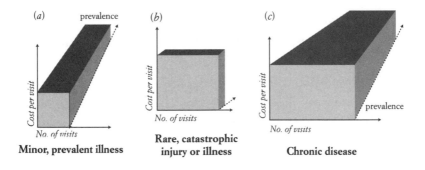

1. Prevalence in the population: Is it common?
2. Cost per interaction with the medical system: Is it costly?
3. Number of visits required to medical-care providers: Is it continuous?

Payer organizations control costs by minimizing how common, costly, and continuous a disease or illness is among their policy holders. The first profile (*a*) shows health-care utilization for a minor, prevalent illness such as a cold or flu, for which the cost per doctor visit is low and the number of visits per person small, yet millions of people are affected. Payer organizations have been able to control the cost of colds and flu by providing free flu vaccines to reduce the number of people who are affected. A rare, catastrophic illness or accident (*b*), such as hemophilia or head injury, affects relatively few people; the cost per doctor visit is high, and the number of visits required is also high. Reducing the cost of interactions with the medical system by establishing, for example, home care instead of hospital care will have a more significant impact on costs than trying to control the prevalence of these more random catastrophes. The acute-care-based medical system we have in the United States was designed to accommodate these minor, prevalent and/or rare, catastrophic illnesses, but chronic disease (*c*), such as diabetes, cancer, or AIDS, does not fit in. These diseases affect large populations that will, for a long time, depend on multiple health-care disciplines in a way that is actuarially difficult to predict. Such is the case with diabetes, which diverges into a complex array of secondary diseases without any predictable or well-defined outcome.

Diabetes is big business for powerful economic, social, and political forces that open and close doors to our treatments and cures. Billions of dollars are made from selling products to the diabetic community. Large diabetes-specific losses are accrued to diabetic people, taxpayers, and the insurance companies left holding our medical policies. During the 1970s and early 1980s, fee-for-service policies, in which insurance companies paid whatever physicians charged, were the standard form of medical coverage. Indemnity abuses were rampant, causing insurance premiums to rise rapidly. It was this time of runaway costs that opened the door to strict payer supervision. Medical inflation grew faster than inflation in the Consumer Price Index. As Lee Iacocca explained it, premiums for employees' health insurance rose more than the cost of steel that went into producing cars. Managed-care organizations showed American companies how to cut costs by buying into health maintenance organizations (HMOs), community-based networks of physicians, hospitals, and other health-care providers. Market forces fueled the growth of managed care, so that by the late 1980s HMOs dominated the health-care system.

The economics imposed by managed care have changed the countenance of caregiver-patient relationships. Patients' choices, formerly the domain of the doctor and patient, are directed by a variety of reimbursement strategies—copayments, deductibles, and outright nonpayment of medical bills. Primary-care physicians act as "gatekeepers" to control the cost of treatments and procedures by restricting access to specialists, so that increasingly diabetics are seen by general practitioners rather than by diabetologists and endocrinologists. Insurance companies seek ways to delay or avoid expensive treatments. Doctors can be subject to losses of income of as much as 30 percent for recommending treatments that are unnecessary in the opinion of the managed-care organizations that have included them in their networks. Practices that fail to demonstrate savings are at risk of being excluded from the networks. These pressures have often meant that diabetic patients are not referred to eye, kidney, heart, and pancreas-transplant specialists until late in the progression of secondary complications. Patients' rights groups have protested the practices of the totalitarian HMOs. Now, out of the extremes of managed care come the more moderate preferred provider organizations (PPOs), which provide greater coverage for people who choose to see doctors out of their network. Today, PPOs have 40 percent more members (105 million) than HMOs (75 million).[13]

In both HMOs and PPOs, reimbursement schemes are not structured to encourage expensive procedures. In this tide pool of warring incentives, it is not surprising that diabetes educators, case managers, and physicians hear little about new medical treatments that are more expensive than traditional diabetes management. The result is that diabetic patients often are unaware of their treatment options. Those who do learn about expensive treatments such as pancreas transplants and insulin pumps often wade through a series of denials and appeals before getting approval from their insurance companies. Many never get approvals.

Concerned about being passed by for promotions or losing out on career opportunities because of health, diabetics often avoid telling their employers they have diabetes. Consequently, when employers negotiate to buy group health policies, they are often unaware of how many of their employees have diabetes, let alone the nature of their health-care needs. Two million people per year are denied health insurance for medical reasons, according to a report written for the Health Care Policy and Research Agency.[14] As we approach the turn

[13]Milt Freudenheim, "(Loosely) Managed Care is in Demand," *New York Times*, September 29, 1998, p. C1.

[14]K. M. Beauregard, "Persons Denied Private Health Insurance Due to Poor Health," Agency for Health Care Policy and Research, Report No. 92-0016, December 1991.

of the century, 58 million Americans have *no* medical coverage. Often people with health problems pay higher or "rated" insurance premiums.[15] For diabetics, the risk of being unemployed, and therefore uninsured, increases as secondary complications and expenses associated with treatment rise. With an ever-increasing prevalence of diabetes (an estimated 800,000 new cases per year), rising costs, and a depleted health-care system, the need to prevent and cure the disease is even more urgent than before.

But the cures to date are expensive. Should we spend $60,000 to $90,000 for a single pancreas transplant? Can the high cost be justified when so many are under- or uninsured? If the issue were purely one of short-term economics, as it is for most insurance companies, the answer may be "No." However, from the individual's perspective the answer should be an unequivocal "Yes." Everyone has the right to pursue the best treatment option available. Insurance companies find it difficult to rationalize the economics of pancreas transplantation within the context of their short-term revenue horizons. The National Institutes of Health, citing the National Cooperative Transplantation Study, believes that the costs of simultaneous pancreas and kidney transplants are exceeded by the costs of four years of dialysis.[16] This opinion was corroborated by Robert Stratta, M.D., the director of

[15]Conrad F. Meier, "How to Implement Kassebaum-Kennedy," Heartland Policy Study (Chicago: Heartland Institute, March 1997).

[16]T. V. Holohan, "Simultaneous Pancreas-Kidney and Sequential Pancreas after Kidney Transplantation," U.S. Public Health Service, Agency for Health Care Policy and Research, Health Technology Assessment, 4:1–53.

pancreas transplantation at the University of Tennessee, in Memphis, who analyzed the relative cost of dialysis, solitary kidney transplants, and simultaneous pancreas and kidney transplants over a four-year period. Simultaneous pancreas and kidney transplants were less expensive than dialysis and, after four years, only $34,800 more expensive than kidney transplants alone.

A five-year analysis of cost, incorporating quality of life and cost per quality-adjusted year, published in the *American Journal of Kidney Diseases*, showed that simultaneous pancreas and kidney transplants are the most cost-effective treatment of diabetic kidney failure. Simultaneous pancreas and kidney transplants (insulin free, dialysis free) were more cost-effective than solitary kidney transplants (insulin dependent, dialysis free), which in turn were more cost-effective than dialysis (insulin dependent, dialysis dependent).[17]

Beyond the economics, pancreas transplantation has helped researchers to understand such things as autoimmunity, beta-cell function, insulin production and secretion, and the process of rejection and how to detect it, indeed have also provided a foundation of knowledge to progress to safer, more efficient, and less costly treatments with cellular replacement. Diabetes has always been managed reactively, with too little sensitivity to the long-term impact of the disease. Consequently we are still living with the temporary solution of day-to-day blood-sugar management. To control the human and economic costs of diabetes, the focus needs

[17]V. Douzdjian, D. Ferrara, G. Silvestri, "Treatment Strategies for Insulin-Dependent Diabetic with ESRD: A Cost Effectiveness Decision Analysis Model." *American Journal of Kidney Diseases* 31, no. 5 (May 1998): 794–802.

to shift to using technology to solve the underlying metabolic defect.

As discussed in Chapter 14, many physicians and scientists over the past twenty-five years have been working to make it possible to cure diabetes with a small mass of insulin-producing cells. Now, some of them are taking their laboratory successes "from the bench to the bedside" with carefully regulated human trials. With proof that diabetes can be cured in large animals using islets and no immunosuppression, we have a similar basis for applying abundant resources to curing diabetes to that which FDR had in the 1930s when he removed the obstacles from the path of eradicating polio. As Dr. Bernhard Hering, who has the most consistent record of success with human islet transplantation to date, says, "There is nothing special or magical about islet transplantation, it just needs to be done. Kidney transplantation is working because 500,000 kidney transplants have been done and lessons have been learned, and have been implemented. Ten thousand pancreas transplants have been done and that is why pancreas transplantation is now very effective. A few more than 300 islet transplants have been done worldwide, not 3,000."[18]

Most laboratory experiments that are conducted to find answers to mechanistic questions are funded by government and private research dollars through an effective system of peer review and selection. Clinical trials require a higher level of committed funding to support a range of tasks including

[18]Bernhard Hering, "Today's Solutions for Diabetes: Islet Transplantaion," paper given at Insulin-Free World Foundation seminar, St. Louis, Mo., May 16, 1998.

patient recruitment, pancreas and tissue acquisition, hospi-
talization costs, surgical fees, medications, and data collection and analysis. Until now, the majority of human islet
transplants have been conducted at six centers: in the United
States in St. Louis, Minneapolis, and Miami; in Europe in
Milan and Giessen; and in Canada in Edmonton, Alberta.
Yet funding has been sporadic. At the end of 1998, the Juvenile Diabetes Foundation funded a new islet research facility
at Harvard University to bring together more than thirty of
the world's finest researchers to focus on diabetes research.
Also in 1998, the National Institutes of Health (NIH) and the
National Institute of Diabetes and Digestive and Kidney Diseases (NIDDK) joined the fight by announcing the establishment of a fully funded transplant program that has as one of
its goals perfecting a cure for diabetes without the need for
ongoing immunosuppression. The program will recruit vol-
unteers (at no cost to diabetic patients) to test new protocols
with pancreas and islet transplants.

At last we have everything required for large-scale islet
transplant trials in humans; multidisciplinary transplant facil-
ities, funding, volunteer patients, surgical staff, transplant
coordinators, high-quality islets, and a backlog of protocols
that are safe to test. But science alone can no more eradicate
diabetes than Jonas Salk, who developed the polio vaccine,
could have purged the world of polio. As Dr. Salk said in a
1991 interview in San Diego, "It was possible to do what I've
done simply because others did see what I saw. . . . If you
don't have the support of others you cannot achieve anything. . . . It's like a cry in the wilderness."[19]

[19]Hall of Science and Exploration, Interview with Jonas Salk, M.D.,
San Diego, California., May 16, 1991.

It has taken a long time to get the ball rolling to cure diabetes, but it *is* rolling. Yet there is still a distance to go to the safe, widespread, low-cost cure that we aspire to, so we need to push like crazy until diabetes is extinct. Tax dollars spent on disease research are shared disproportionately among major diseases relative to the number of people affected, economic cost, and death rates. How much and how fast funding, research and policy are applied to cure diabetes is a direct function of our demand. Research funding is subject to how effectively advocates lobby for their particular disease. These comments should not be construed to minimize the severity of any disease, as I am pointing, not to the disease itself, but to the politics beyond. Take, for example, funding for prostate versus breast cancer. Although they both cause about the same number of deaths per year, funding for breast cancer is five times higher than that for prostate cancer. According to an article in *Business Week* by Gary Becker, the 1992 Nobel laureate in medicine, breast cancer research is "so much better funded partly because sufferers are better organized for political activity. Men have tended to keep quiet about their prostate cancers." Becker notes that AIDS research receives four times the funding of breast cancer, and more than twenty times the funds of prostate cancer. "The political effectiveness of AIDS activists surely helps explain why a much larger chunk of the federal budget is allocated to AIDS research than to other terrible and painful ailments," Becker writes.[20]

---

[20]Gary Becker, "The Painful Political Truth about Medical Research," Economic Viewpoint, *Business Week*, July 29, 1996. p. 18

Impact of Diabetes Relative to Breast Cancer and AIDS

Disease	No. afflicted	Annual Deaths	Direct Cost	Govt. research budget
Breast cancer + AIDS	3.35 million	75,000	16.9 billion	$2.1 billion
Diabetes	16 million	180,000	91.1 billion	$316 million

Source: American Diabetes Association "Dear Candidate for Congress Letter, *Diabetes Advocate*, September 1998, p. 3.

The government spends $1,700 on AIDS research for each person with AIDS, but less than $20 on diabetes research for each person with diabetes. In 1997, $13 *billion* was spent to try to cure diseases, but only 2.5% of that, $316 *million*, was spent on diabetes research.[21] Advocates for AIDS and cancer encourage financial and political support with well-publicized reports of each research success and imminent breakthrough in treatments for their diseases, yet have remained staunchly focused on cures. We send mixed messages about diabetes. In an effort to encourage optimism and confidence, diabetes magazines and educational materials show images of active, healthy people "managing their condition" with a "no problem" attitude. Pharmaceutical companies use images and slogans of smiling diabetic people holding their products, the symbols of diabetes—syringes, blood-glucose-monitoring equipment, glucose tablets. But the disease itself is not revealed.

[21]American Diabetes Association, *Diabetes Advocate*, September 1998, p. 3.

The public perception of diabetes is influenced by our personal testimonies. We have portrayed a disease that is no more than a minor inconvenience. It is little wonder that when things go wrong, we are accused of noncompliance, mismanagement, and "cheating" on diets. Diabetic complications have served as a line of demarcation between those who are proud to speak out and those who hide. People who are doing well with diabetes, who are congratulated and respected for their ability to control their disease, become the faces that peer out of the pages of articles, advertisements, and diabetes education brochures.

By showing the world only the happy face, and not the tragic disease beneath, we are endorsing the prevailing philosophy of tolerating, rather than curing, diabetes. For policymakers, philanthropists, employers, and the public to feel compelled to cure diabetes, they need to understand that diabetes is costly for society; that those costs are rising; that it is pervasive and the incidence is accelerating; that it is soul destroying; that there is still no cure; and, above all, that diabetes *is curable*. There needs to be a fundamental shift in the way diabetes is viewed. The following letter, which we received at the Insulin-Free World Foundation, provides an example of the asymmetry between letting the world think that diabetes is not a problem and wanting a cure:

> I am a diabetic who has been living with the condition for over 17 years. I have been impressed by the widespread publicity initiated by the "Diabetes Stinks. Know Your Options" billboard campaign in California. They are indeed in very prominent locations, and it seems that everyone I know has noticed them. HOWEVER, I would

like to express my concern over the message that is being sent by those billboards:

1) The prominent message is indeed true, BUT it invokes an unnecessarily negative feeling towards the condition. I have endured some of the complications of diabetes, and I think a more positive and inspiring message would be far more effective.

2) Even more alarming is the message that this sends to non-diabetics. Every diabetic has had the difficult task of explaining the condition to other people and encouraging them to feel comfortable and not to be overly worried about it. The negative message I think does the opposite.

I am very ambivalent about sending my concerns to you, because few people could be more interested about a cure or improved treatment of diabetes than I am!

We have phenomenal potential in our hands, because we know the whole truth about diabetes. Just as FDR did with his disease, we must wage war on diabetes using public policy, our votes, nonprofit organizations, social awareness, pharmaceutical companies, medical researchers, doctors, nurses, government agencies, and the media. Polio was abolished by people—through acts of will and persistence. That is what it will take to cure diabetes, too.

There is no good time to become diabetic, but the person being diagnosed today has every reason to believe that diabetes will *not* last a lifetime, and that secondary complications are no more than an ugly chapter in the history of the disease. The momentum to cure diabetes is building as it absorbs the energy of the "independent tributaries, springs and rains" of research that feed it. Myriad paths of research are gaining momentum and converging: islet isolation and preservation;

immune tolerance; human islet transplantation, encapsulation, and xenotransplantation; islet-cell proliferation and regeneration; stem cell engineering; and genetic engineering. When I was diagnosed in 1970, diabetes was a life sentence and insulin was something I would need forever to survive; now I am insulin free. The sense of excitement and renewed energy is palpable as the diabetic community hears that we already have ways to overcome diabetes. The U.S. government has now proved it is committed to curing diabetes by allocating funds and resources to implement human islet-transplant trials and to pursuing new immunology protocols that will benefit pancreas recipients as well. Private funds are flowing into institutions whose single-minded mission is to cure diabetes. All we have to do is to keep pushing the ball, to seek information about our options, to demand that our health insurance policies allow for those options, and to let the world know that curing diabetes is a worthy mission.

I am reminded of a story I heard once about a little boy in a tribal village who thought he had found the perfect way to trick one of the wise elders. Clasping his hands tightly behind his back, he approached the elder and said, "Tell me, is the bird in my hand alive or dead?" He thought to himself, "I've got him either way. If he says the bird is dead, I'll open my hands and the bird will fly away, and I will say, 'You are wrong, the bird is alive!' But if on the other hand he says the bird is alive, I'll close my hands more tightly and the bird will be dead." The elder thought to himself for just a minute, then said, "The bird is in your hands. Whether the bird lives or dies is up to you."

Appendix

Pancreas and Islet Transplant Centers

United States by State

University of Alabama at
  Birmingham
Department of Surgery
Division of Transplantation
701 South 19th Street
Birmingham, AL 35294

University of Arizona
  Medical Center
Department of Transplant
  Service
1501 N. Campbell Avenue
Tucson, AZ 85724

University of Arkansas
  Hospital
Department of Surgery
4301 West Markham Street
Box 520
Little Rock, AR 77205-7199

California Pacific Medical
  Center
Transplant Service
P.O. Box 7999
2340 Clay Street, Suite 417
San Francisco, CA 94115

Loma Linda University
   Medical Center
Transplant Institute
11234 Anderson Street
Suite 1405
Loma Linda, CA 92354

Southern California
   Transplantation Institute
Transplantation Center
4500 Brockton Avenue
Suite 103
Riverside, CA 92501

St. Vincent Medical Center
Department of
   Transplantation
2131 West Third Street
Los Angeles, CA 90057

Stanford Medical Center
Department of Surgery
750 Welch Road
Suite 200
Palo Alto, CA 94304-5785

Sutter Memorial Hospital
Transplant Services
5151 F Street
Sacramento, CA 95819-3295

UCLA School of Medicine
Center for Health Sciences
Department of Surgery
10833 LeConte Avenue
Los Angeles, CA 90024-
6904

University of California,
   Davis Medical Center
Transplant Clinic
2315 Stockton Blvd.
House Staff Facility
Sacramento, CA 95817

University of California,
   San Francisco
Transplant Service
Moffitt Hospital, Room 884
P.O. Box 0116
San Francisco, CA
   94143-0116

University of California,
   San Diego Medical Center
Department of Surgery
200 West Arbor Drive
San Diego, CA 92103-8401

Porter Adventist Hospital
Transplant Service
2535 S. Downing Street
Suite 380
Denver, CO 80210-5850

Presbyterian/St. Luke's
    Medical Center
Transplant Program
1719 East 19th Avenue
Denver, CO 80218

University of Colorado
    Health Sciences Center
Department of Transplant
    Surgery
4200 East Ninth Avenue
Box C-318
Denver, CO 80212

Hartford Transplant
    Associates
Northeast Organ
    Procurement &
    Transplant Services
85 Seymour Street
Suite 319
Hartford, CT 06102

Yale New Haven Hospital
Division of Organ
    Transplantation
333 Cedar Street
New Haven, CT 06510

Georgetown University
    Medical Center
Transplant Center
3800 Reservoir Road, NW
PHC Room 4004
Washington, DC 20007

Walter Reed Army
    Medical Center
Organ Transplant Service
WD48, WRAMC
6825 Georgia Avenue, NW
Washington, DC
    20307-5001

Washington Hospital
    Center
Transplant Service
110 Irving Street NW
Washington, DC 20010

University of Florida,
 Shands Hospital
Department of Transplant
 Surgery
P.O. Box 100286
1600 SW Archer Rd.
Gainesville, FL 32610-0286

University of Miami
 Transplant Program
Professional Arts Center,
Suite 605
1150 NW 14th Street
Miami, FL 33136

Emory University Hospital
Department of Surgery
Transplant Division
1364 Clifton Road, NE
Suite H-124
Atlanta, GA 30322

Medical College of Georgia
Department of Surgery
1120 15th Street
Transplant Office,
 Room BA 4407
Augusta, GA 30912-4092

St. Francis Medical Center
Department of Surgery
2230 Liliha Street
Honolulu, HI 96817

University of Iowa
 Hospital and Clinics
Department of Surgery
Transplant Service
200 Hawkins Drive
Iowa City, IA 52242-1086

Northwestern University
 Medical School
Division of Transplantation
303 E. Superior Street
Passavant Pavilion,
 Suite 528
Chicago, IL 60611-3053

Rush–Presbyterian
 St. Luke's Medical Center
University Transplant
 Program
1725 W. Harrison,
 Suite 161
Chicago, IL 60612

Southern Illinois University
Memorial Medical Center
Transplant Service
701 First Street
Springfield, IL 62781

University of Chicago
Section of Transplant
  Surgery
5841 S. Maryland Avenue
M/C 5026
Chicago, IL 60637

University of Illinois
  Hospital
Department of Surgery
840 South Wood Street
Room 402, M/C 958
Chicago, IL 60612-7322

Indiana University
  Medical Center
Organ Transplant Center
550 N. University Blvd.
Indianapolis, IN
  46202-5250

Via Christie–St. Francis
  Medical Center
Department of
  Transplantation
929 North St. Francis
Wichita, KS 67214

Jewish Hospital
Department of Surgery
217 E. Chestnut Street
Louisville, KY 40202-1886

University of Kentucky
  Medical Center
Transplant Department
800 Rose Street
Lexington, KY 40536-0084

Louisiana State University
Regional Transplant Center
Department of Surgery
3315 Virginia Avenue
Shreveport, LA 71103

Ochsner Foundation
  Hospital
Multi-Organ Transplant
  Center
1514 Jefferson Highway,
  BH 321
New Orleans, LA
  70121-2483

Transplant Institute of
New Orleans
Department of Surgery
3535 Bienville Street
Suite 225
New Orleans, LA 70119

Tulane University Medical
Center
Department of Surgery
1430 Tulane Avenue
New Orleans, LA 70112

Baystate Medical Center
Department of
Transplantation
759 Chestnut Street
Springfield, MA
01199-0001

Beth Israel Hospital
Division of Transplantation
330 Brookline Avenue
Boston, MA 02215

Massachusetts General
Hospital
Harvard Medical School
Gray 505
55 Fruit Street
Boston, MA 02114

New England Deaconess
Hospital
Division of Organ
Transplant
185 Pilgrim Road
Boston, MA 02215

University of
Massachusetts Medical
Center
Department of Transplant
Surgery
55 Lake Avenue North,
53-709
Worcester, MA 01655

Johns Hopkins Medical
Institute
Department of Transplant
Surgery
600 North Wolfe Street
Baltimore, MD 21287-0005

University of Maryland
Medical Center
Department of Surgery
Division of Organ
Transplantation
29 S. Greene Street,
Suite 200
Baltimore, MD 21201

Henry Ford Hospital
Department of Transplant
  Surgery
2799 West Grand Blvd.
Detroit, MI 48202-2689

St. John Hospital and
  Medical Center
Transplant Specialty Center
22101 Moross Road
Professional Building II
Suite 174
Detroit, MI 48236

University of Michigan
  Medical Center
Division of Transplant
  Surgery
2926 Taubman Center,
  Box 0331
1500 E. Medical Center
  Drive
Ann Arbor, MI 48109-0331

Fairview–University
  Medical Center
Transplant Center
516 Delaware Street, SE
Minneapolis, MN 55455

Mayo Clinic
Department of Surgery
Eisenburg L-G
200 First Street, SW
Rochester, MN 55905

St. Louis University
  Hospital
Abdominal Organ
  Transplantation
3635 Vista Ave. at
  Grand Blvd.
P.O. Box 15250
St. Louis, MO 63110-0250

Carolinas Medical Center
Transplant Center
P.O. Box 32861
Charlotte, NC 28203

Duke University Medical
  Center
Department of Surgery
Box 3510
Durham, NC 27710

University of North
Carolina
School of Medicine
Department of Surgery
3010 Old Clinic Building
CB 7210
Chapel Hill, NC
27599-7210

Nebraska Health System
Kidney/Pancreas
Transplant Services
Clarkson Hospital
987555 Nebraska Medical
Center
Omaha, NE 68198-7555

Our Lady of Lourdes
Hospital
Transplant Department
1600 Haddon Avenue
Camden, NJ 08103-3117

St. Barnabas Medical
Center
Transplant Department
East Wing, Suite 303
Old Short Hills Road
Livingston, NJ 07039

University Medical Center
of Southern Nevada
Transplant Services
1800 West Charleston Blvd.
Las Vegas, NV 89102

Albany Medical Center
Hospital
Department of Surgery
47 New Scotland Avenue
Albany, NY 12208

Columbia Presbyterian
Medical Center
Department of Surgery
161 Fort Washington
Avenue
New York, NY 10032

Mount Sinai Medical
Center
Transplant Division
Box 1104
New York, NY 10029

New York University
Medical Center
Transplantation Surgery
530 First Avenue, Suite 6A
New York, NY 10016

Strong Memorial Hospital
Department of Transplant
  Surgery
601 Elmwood Avenue
Rochester, NY 14642-8410

SUNY Health Science
  Center, Brooklyn
Division of Organ
  Transplantation
450 Clarkson Avenue,
  Box 40
Brooklyn, NY 11203-2098

SUNY Health Sciences
  Center, Syracuse
Department of Surgery
750 East Adams Street
Syracuse, NY 13210

Cleveland Clinic
  Foundation
General Surgery
Desk A110
9500 Euclid Avenue
Cleveland, OH 44195-5241

Ohio State University
  Hospital
Department of Surgery
Division of Transplantation
Room 345 Means Hall
1654 Upham Drive
Columbus, OH 43210-1228

University Hospitals of
  Cleveland
Department of Surgery
Transplant Division
11100 Euclid Avenue
Cleveland, OH 44106

University of Cincinnati
  Medical Center
Department of Surgery
Transplantation Division
P.O. Box 670558
231 Bethesda Avenue
Cincinnati, OH 45267-0558

Oklahoma Transplant
  Institute
Pancreas Transplant
  Division
3300 NW Expressway
Oklahoma City, OK
  73112-4418

University of Oklahoma
Hospital
Transplant Services
Room 5E190
800 NE 13th Street
Oklahoma City, OK 73104

Oregon Health Sciences
University
Department of Clinical
Transplant
3505 SW Veterans Hospital
Road
Portland, OR 97201

Albert Einstein Medical
Center
Department of Transplant
Surgery
Suite 505
5401 Old York Road
Philadelphia, PA 19141

Allegheny University
Hospital
Division of Transplant
Broad & Vine Streets
Mail Stop 417
Philadelphia, PA 19102-
1192

Pennsylvania State
University Hospital
Milton S. Hershey Medical
Center
Department of Surgery
Section of Transplantation
500 University Drive, P.O.
Box 850
Hershey, PA 17033

Presbyterian University
Hospital of Pittsburgh
Department of Surgery
Division of Transplant
4 Falk Clinic
3601 Fifth Avenue
Pittsburgh, PA 15213

University of Pennsylvania
Hospital
Department of Multi-Organ
Transplant
3400 Spruce Street
Philadelphia, PA 19104-4283

Medical University of South
Carolina
Department of Surgery
171 Ashley Avenue
Charleston, SC 29425

Johnson City Medical
 Center Hospital
Transplant Services
408 N. State off Franklin
 Road, Suite 46
Johnson City, TN
 37604-6094

University of Tennessee
 Memphis
Division of Transplantation
956 Court Avenue
Suite A202
Memphis, TN 38163

Vanderbilt Transplant
 Center
912 Oxford House
Nashville, TN 37232-4750

Methodist Hospital
Baylor College of Medicine
Multi-Organ Transplant
 Center
6565 Fannin Street,
 Suite 447
Houston, TX 77030

Methodist Medical Center
Transplant Service
P.O. Box 655999
1441 N. Beckley Blvd.
Dallas, TX 75265-5999

Parkland Memorial
 Hospital
Transplant Clinic
5201 Harry Hines Blvd.
Dallas, TX 75235-7747

San Antonio Regional
 Hospital
Renal/Pancreas Program
8026 Floyd Curl Drive
3 West
San Antonio, TX 78229

University of Texas at
 Houston
Division of Immunology
 and Transplantation
Health Science Center
6431 Fannin Street,
 Suite 6-252
Houston, TX 77030

University of Texas Health
Science Center
Department of Surgery
7703 Floyd Curl Drive
San Antonio, TX
78284-7842

University of Texas Medical
Branch
Department of Surgery
Route 0262
301 University Boulevard
Galveston, TX 77555-0262

LDS Hospital
Department of
Transplantation
8th Avenue and C Street
Salt Lake City, UT 84143

Inova Fairfax Hospital
Inova Transplant Center
3300 Gallows Road
Falls Church, VA 22046

Medical College of Virginia
Hospital
Division of Vascular and
Transplant Surgery
Box 980057
Richmond, VA 23298

University of Virginia
Department of Surgery
P.O. Box 10005
Charlottesville, VA
22906-0005

Swedish Hospital
Pancreas Organ Transplant
Program
1120 Cherry Street,
Suite 400
Seattle, WA 98104-2196

University of Washington
Medical Center
Transplant Services
1959 NE Pacific Street
Box 356174
Seattle, WA 98195-6174

Virginia Mason Medical
Center
Division of Renal/Pancreas
Transplant
1100 Ninth Avenue, C7-N
Seattle, WA 98111

Froedtert Memorial
  Lutheran Hospital
Medical College of
  Wisconsin
Organ Procurement Office
9200 West Wisconsin
  Avenue
Milwaukee, WI 53226

University of Wisconsin
  Hospital and Clinics
Division of Organ
  Transplantation
H4/785 Clinical Science
  Center
600 Highland Avenue
Madison, WI 53792-7375

Internationally by Country

Hospital Italiano de Buenos
  Aires
Pancreas and Islet
  Transplant Program
Gascon 450
Buenos Aires 1181
Argentina

Australian National
  Pancreas Transplant Unit
Westmead Hospital
Westmead, NSW 2145
Sydney
Australia

University of Innsbruck
Department of
  Transplantation
Anichstrasse 35
A-6020 Innsbruck
Austria

Catholic University of
  Leuven
Transplant Surgery
UZ Gasthuisberg
Herestraat 49
Leuven 3000
Belgium

Universitéde Liège
Centre Hospitalier
Boireau de Transplantation
Domaine Universitaire du
  Sart-Tilman
1 B.35-4000
Belgium

University Hospital
Department of Surgery
B-9000 Gent
Belgium

Universite de Brussels
Erasme-Clinique
Nephrology/Dialysis/
  Transplant Department
808 Rte. de Lennik
B-1070 Brussels
Belgium

University of Louvain
  Medical School
Department of Pancreatic
  Transplantation
Saint Luc Hospital
10 Hippocrate Avenue
B-1200 Brussels
Belgium

Beneficencia Portuguesa
  Hospital
Clinica De Especialidades
  Cirurgicas
Rua Maestro Cardim 377
Cj.75
Paraiso CEP 01323-001
Sao Paulo
Brazil

British Columbia
  Transplant Society
4th Floor, East Tower
555 West 12th Avenue
Vancouver, BC V5Z 3X7
Canada

Hopital de Notre Dame
Laboratoire de Nephrologie
1560 Sherbrooke Est
Montreal, PQ H2L 4M1
Canada

Queen Elizabeth II Health
  Sciences Centre
Transplant Program
1278 Tower Road
Halifax, NS B3H 2Y9
Canada

University Hospital
Multi-organ Transplant
  Service
339 Windermere Road
London, ON N6A 5A5
Canada

University of Alberta
  Hospital
Department of Surgery
204.37 Walter Mackenzie
  Centre
Edmonton, AB T6G 2B7
Canada

University of Toronto
Multi-Organ Transplant
  Program
200 Elizabeth Street
10 Norman Urquhart Wing,
Room 114
Toronto, ON M5G 2C4
Canada

Unidad de Trasplantes
Clinica las Condes
Lo Fontecilla 441
Santiago
Chile

Clinic San Pedro Claver
Department of Surgery
Transplant Service
Carrera 30 Avenue de Las
  Americas
Bogata
Colombia

Hospital Calderon Guardia
Department of Surgery
Aranjuez
P.O. Box 3679
San Jose
Costa Rica

Institute for Clinical and
  Experimental Medicine
Diabetes Department
Videnska 800
14000 Prague 4
Czech Republic

Odense University Hospital
Department of Nephrology
DK-5000 Odense
Denmark

Centre Hospitalier
  Hautepiere
Transplant Unit
Avenue Molière
Strasbourg CEDEX 67098
France

Centre Hospitalier,
  University Nancy
Hospital de Brabois
Department of Nephrology
54511 Vandoeuvre
Nancy CEDEX
France

Hôpital Edouard Herriot
Urology and Transplant
  Surgery
5 Place d'Arsonval
Lyon 69003
France

Hôpital Leannec
Diabetologie-Nutrition-
  Transplantation
42 Rue de Sevres
Paris 75007
France

Hôpital Pitie, Salpetrière
Department of Urology
47 et 83 Bd. de l'Hôpital
Paris, CEDEX 13, 75851
France

Nantes University Hospital
Nephrology and Clinical
  Immunology
30 Bd. Jean Monet
Nantes 44000
France

University Hospital
  Lapeyronie
Department of
  Transplantation
371 Avenue de Soyen
  Giraud
Montpelier 34295
France

University Hospital of
  Bicetre
Department of Nephrology
78 Av. du General Lecierc
Kremlin-Bicetre, CEDEX
  94275
France

Humboldt-University,
Virchow-Klinikum
Department of Surgery
Hugustenburger Platz 1
Berlin D-13353
Germany

Justus-Liebig-University of
Giessen
3rd Medical Department
and Policlinic
University of Giessen,
Rodthohl 6
Giessen D-35385
Germany

Ludwig-Maximilians-
Universität München
Klinikum
Transplantation Schirurgie
Marchioninistrasse 15
München D-81366
Germany

Medical University of
Luebeck
Department of Surgery
Ratzeburger Allee 160
Luebeck D-2400
Germany

Universität Klinikum Essen
Department of General
Surgery
Hufelandstrasse 55
Essen D-45142
Germany

Albert-Ludwigs-Universität
Hospital
Department of Surgery
Section of Transplantation
Hugstetter Strasse 55
Freilburg D-79106
Germany

University Hospital of
Marburg
Department of Internal
Medicine
Baldingcr Strasse
Marburg D-35033
Germany

Universität Klinikum
Eppendorf
Department of General
Surgery
Martinistrasse 52
Hamburg D-20246
Germany

University of Bochum,
Knappschaftskrankenhaus
Department of Surgery
In Der Schornau 23-25
Bochum D-44892
Germany

University of Rostock
Department of Transplant
Surgery
Schillingallee 35
Rostock D-18057
Germany

University of Saarland
Department of Surgery
Hamburg D-66421
Germany

University of Tuebingen
Department of Surgery
Hoppe-Seyler Strasse 3
Transplant Center
Tuebingen D-72076
Germany

University of Wuerzburg
Department of Surgery
Josef-Schneider-Strasse 2
Wuerzburg D-97080
Germany

University Ulm Klinikum
Department of Surgery II
Steinhovelstrasse 9
Ulm D-89075
Germany

Albert Szent–Gyorgyi
Medical University
Department of Surgery
P.O. Box 464
Pesci u. 4
Szeged H-6701
Hungary

Beaumont Hospital
Department of
Transplantation
P.O. Box 1297
Beaumont Road
Dublin 9
Ireland

Beilinson Medical Centre
Department of Organ
Transplantation
Zabotinski 66
Petah Tikva 49100
Israel

Instituto San Raffaele
Ospedale
Department of Surgery
Via Olgettina 60
I-20132 Milano
Italy

Ospedale Reg
"Monoblocco–San
Martino"
University of Genova
Department of Surgery
Viale Benedetto XV, 6
I-16132 Genova
Italy

Treviso General Hospital
Transplant Center
Piazza Ospedale
I-31100 Treviso
Italy

University di Genova
Ospedas San Martino
Clinica Chirurgica Generale
Via le Benedetto XV, 6
I-16132 Genova
Italy

University di Padova
1st di Chir Generale II
Ospedale Guistinianeo
Via Guistinianeo 2
I-35128 Padova
Italy

University of Perugia
DIMISEM
Via E. dal Pozzo
I-06126 Perugia
Italy

University of Verona
Department of Surgery
I-37134 Verona
Italy

Especialidades Ctr. Medicine
Nacional Siglo XXI
Transplant Unit
Av. Cuauhtemoc 330
Col Doctores
Heriberto Frias 112-8
CP 03020
Mexico City DF 06720
Mexico

Hospital de Especialidades
71
Instituto Mexicano del
Seguro Soc.
Transplant Unit/
Department of Surgery
Blvd. Revolucion y Calle 27
Torreon, Coahuila 27000
Mexico

Academisch Ziekenhuis
Transplant Surgery
P.O. Box 9600
2300 RC Leiden
The Netherlands

University Hospital
Groningen
Department of Surgery
Hanzeplein 1
9713 GZ Groningen
The Netherlands

University of Oslo
Rikshospitalet
The National Hospital
Department of Surgery
Pilestredet 32
N-0027 Oslo
Norway

First Affiliated Hospital–
Henan Medical University
Department of Surgery
Division of Pancreatic
Transplantation
40 Da Xue Rd.
Postcode 450052
Zhengzhou, Henan
Peoples Republic of China

Germans Trias I Pujol
Department of Nephrology
Crta de Canyet
E-08916 Badalona
Spain

Hospital Clinic 1 Provincial
De Barcelona
Edifici D'Urgencies
Planta 1-Despatx #4
Villarroel, 170
E-08036 Barcelona
Spain

Hospital Regional Carlos
Haya
Coordinacion de
Transplantes
Avda Carlos Haya s/n
E-29010 Malaga
Spain

Hospital Universitario San
   Carlos
Ciudad Univeritaria
Departamento di Cirurgia
Ciudad Universitaria
E-28040 Madrid
Spain

Karolinska Institute
Huddinge Hospital
Department of Transplant
   Surgery
S-14186 Stockholm
Sweden

Malmo University Hospital,
   Lund University
Department of
   Vascular/Renal Disease
Transplant Unit
S. Forstadsgatan 101
S-20502 Malmo
Sweden

Sahlgrenska University
   Hospital
Department of Surgery,
   Division of Transplant
Liver/Vascular Surgery
FACK3
S-41345 Gothenburg
Sweden

University Hospital
   Uppsala
Department of Transplant
   Surgery
Unit 70TD
S-75085 Uppsala
Sweden

University Hospital Geneva
Department of Surgery,
   Transplant Unit
24 Rue Micheli-du-Crest
CH-1211 Geneva 14
Switzerland

University Hospital of
   Zurich
Department of Surgery
Ramistrasse 100
CH-8091 Zurich
Switzerland

Cardiff Royal Infirmary
Department of Transplant
   Surgery
Newport Road
Cardiff
Wales CF2 1SZ
United Kingdom

Guys and St. Thomas'
  Hospital
Pancreas Transplantation
Department of Tissue
  Typing
New Guy's House, Floor 3
London SE1 9RT
United Kingdom

Oxford Radcliffe Hospital
Oxford Transplant Center
The Churchill
Oxford OX3 7LJ
United Kingdom

Royal Liverpool &
  Broadgreen University
Renal Transplant Unit
Link Unit 9C
Prescott Street
Liverpool L7 8XP
United Kingdom

St. Mary's Hospital
Transplant Unit
Praed Street
London W2 1NY
United Kingdom

University of Leicester
Department of Surgery
Leicester LE2 7LX
United Kingdom

Institute for Endocrinology
Diabetes Centre
Dr. Subotica 13
11000 Belgrade
Yugoslavia

Insulin-Free World Foundation

To stay abreast of advances in treatments and cures for diabetes, become a member of the Insulin-Free World Foundation, the nonprofit organization founded by Deb Butterfield in 1996. Benefits of membership include:

- Annual subscription to *Insulin-Free*TIMES
- Five-star, award-winning Web site
- Access to an established network in the diabetic community
- Invitations to seminars
- Awareness campaigns
- Discounts on Insulin-Free World merchandise
- Knowing that you are a part of the solution

For more information, contact the Insulin-Free World Foundation at:

Insulin-Free World Foundation
788 Office Parkway
St. Louis, MO 63141

Tel: 1-888-RING-IFW or 314-468-2440
Fax: 314-468-2444

Visit us on-line at www.insulin-free.org.

The Insulin-Free World Foundation is a nonprofit charitable organization that relies on membership fees and donations for its operation. It is exempt from U.S. Federal Income Taxes under Section 501(C)(3) of the Internal Revenue Code and qualifies for the maximum contribution deduction as allowed by law.